A WORLD WAR II
FLIGHT SURGEON'S STORY

A WORLD WAR II
FLIGHT SURGEON'S STORY

S. CARLISLE MAY
FOREWORD BY MARTIN K. A. MORGAN

PELICAN PUBLISHING COMPANY
GRETNA 2015

The word "Pelican" and the depiction of a pelican are trademarks of Pelican Publishing Company, Inc., and are registered in the U.S. Patent and Trademark Office.

Library of Congress Cataloging-in-Publication Data

May, S. Carlisle.
  A World War II flight surgeon's story / by S. Carlisle May ; foreword by Martin K. A. Morgan.
    pages cm
  Includes bibliographical references and index.
    ISBN 978-1-4556-2048-7 (hardcover : alk. paper) — ISBN 978-1-4556-2049-4 (e-book) 1. Myhr, Lamb B. (Lamb Bolton), 1917-2008. 2. United States. Army Air Forces. 50th Troop Carrier Squadron—Biography. 3. World War, 1939-1945—Medical care—United States. 4. Physicians--United States—Biography. 5. World War, 1939-1945--Aerial operations. I. Title.
  D790.264.M49 2015
  940.54'7573--dc23

                                                       2014044488

Printed in the United States of America
Published by Pelican Publishing Company, Inc.
1000 Burmaster Street, Gretna, Louisiana 70053

In loving memory of my brother, Glenn "Bo" Myhr Plummer, Jr. I'm so glad we shared a love of history. I miss you daily.

Contents

Foreword

In recent years the history of the men and women who fought in World War II has been largely dominated by the voices of those who served at the tip of the spear — the warriors who engaged the enemy in direct action. Although their personal accounts and memoirs, focusing on the experience of combat, have always been popular, they nevertheless provide only a narrow account of wartime service. Those who served in support roles or who were otherwise not directly in the line of fire experienced service during the Second World War in ways that, although slightly less exciting, nevertheless broaden and enlighten our understanding of the conflict.

In the pages that follow, S. Carlisle May recounts the personal experiences of one such individual. As an officer and flight surgeon in the Ninth Air Force's Troop Carrier Command, Lamb Bolton Myhr witnessed firsthand some of the most significant moments of the war in the African/ Middle Eastern/ European theater of operations. From Morocco to the Rhine River, he was a part of each campaign the US Ninth Air Force flew and fought. The author has organized Myhr's letters, photographs, and documents into a narrative revealing not just important aspects of military history but also aspects of the social and cultural history of the Second World War that tell us much about what it took to keep a squadron functioning as an effective team. The officers and men of Myhr's 50th Troop Carrier Squadron moved from one austere duty station to another so that they could go to war in unarmed and unarmored aircraft that were mission critical to Allied victory. Without them, crucial supplies could not have reached the troops who needed them, and airborne operations in Sicily, Italy, Normandy, Holland, and Germany would not have been possible.

Lamb Myhr's World War II story starts when he joins the Army in 1942 and then follows him from Randolph Field near San Antonio, Texas, to Bowman Field in Louisville, Kentucky, and on to Sedalia Army Airfield in Warrensburg, Missouri. It continues in May 1943 when he deploys overseas with the squadron's air echelon in an 8,580-mile journey beginning at Morrison Field in West Palm Beach, Florida, and continuing on to Puerto Rico, Brazil, Ascension Island, Dakar, West Africa, and finally on to Berguent Airfield near Jerada in eastern Morocco. Captain Myhr's squadron ultimately flies from airfields in Tunisia, Sicily, England, and France before VE Day. During this time, he treats everything from burns to VD, and even delivers a baby while the squadron is in Tunisia. In all, his experiences offer a unique perspective of the Second World War in North Africa, the Mediterranean, and Northwest Europe— the kind of perspective that will only become more useful to historians as veterans of the Second World War continue to recede from living memory.

Martin K. A. Morgan
Author/ Historian
Covington, Louisiana

Acknowledgements

This book was a labor of love and learning. There are a number of people that I need to say a few words about.

I cannot say enough how much I appreciate Maranda Gilmore, archivist for the Air Force Historical Research Agency, for the help she provided in finding reports and support information that was invaluable in structuring this book. I also appreciate Marilyn Phar for her help in finding WWII veterans willing to read my manuscript.

Thank you Marty Morgan for writing the foreword. Your knowledge and expert opinion add a stamp of approval that few could give. I'm glad I can call you a friend.

To Joe Lawrence, who read and offered insight. I appreciate your help. Also, thanks for your love and support of the veterans of WWII.

I would like to thank my Tuesday-night critique group— Claudia McCormick, Lisa Folsom, Eleanor Ford, and Paul Franz. You have read, made suggestions, re-read and supported me throughout the writing of this book. I might have been able to do it without you, but it sure was an easier road having you with me.

I can't say enough how grateful I am to Lisa Folsom for reading the second and third time with a fine-tooth comb. You made my work shine. Debbie and Bill Kaufman, thanks for every missing comma. They are all appreciated.

To my sister-in-law, Jeanie, who was married to my

brother, to whom this book is dedicated. I'm grateful for your love and friendship. I couldn't have asked for a better sister. To Jeanie and Bo's children: Katie, Anna, Becky, and Dallas. I see your father in each of you daily; he would be proud of you.

To my mother, I would like to say thank you. You have always been supportive and a great cheerleader. I love you.

I couldn't write day and night and still survive without my family — Drew, Mary Beth, Joseph, Zach, and Nick. I can't leave out the love of my life and husband, Andy, the WWII buff, who helped me talk issues through and made suggestions. I love you all!

Introduction

A World War II Flight Surgeon's Story came about during an afternoon swim on a hot summer day. My brother Bo and I were floating in inner tubes in the lake talking. Our discussion turned to the fact that our great-uncle Lamb, the younger brother of our grandmother on our father's side, was getting older.

We—our family—had always been interested in history. Bo was particularly fascinated with war history. Uncle Lamb had never said much in front of us about his time serving in WWII. The only time I can remember him answering any questions was when we were in our teens and he was at our house for a visit.

Bo and I decided that day in the lake that we needed to see if Uncle Lamb would talk to us about his WWII experiences. Bo would ask the questions, and I would act as secretary. I thought that the information should at least be written down for the family to have. We made plans then to make a trip to East Tennessee during the 2001 Thanksgiving holidays to interview Uncle Lamb.

Just weeks after those plans were made, my brother died in an accident. Talking to Uncle Lamb went by the wayside for a number of years; I couldn't bring myself to do the interview without Bo. Four years after my brother's death, I decided I had to do the interview, knowing I would regret it if I didn't. After speaking to Uncle Lamb, I realized that people outside of my family should also have the opportunity to hear about his experiences during the war. I needed to tell Uncle Lamb's story in book form, and I would dedicate it to Bo.

Uncle Lamb served in the Ninth Air Force of the Army Air Forces. As I read through the war dairy of his squadron, the 50th Troop Carrier Squadron of the IX Troop Carrier Command (TCC), I became familiar with the names of the pilots and crewmembers. Reading the different accounts, I begin to feel like I knew these men. One name stuck out to me in particular because I have a friend with the same last name. I'd "met" the pilot with the last name Dunagan in Africa and later read of his death on D-Day. By that time I had become emotionally involved with the man and was saddened when I read of his death. If I felt that way more than sixty years later from just reading old accounts of the IX TCC, I can only imagine how deeply it must have hurt when Lamb lost a man or a plane full of men.

Additional Stories about Lamb

While going through a lard tin full of old letters that I had inherited from my grandmother, Lamb's older sister, I discovered letters Uncle Lamb had written home to his mother. Most of them have been shared in full in this book. When Lamb writes about his concern for "the boy" or with a request to tell him hi, Uncle Lamb is referring to my father, who lived in the same house with Uncle Lamb during his college and medical-school years.

Some years after the war Uncle Lamb was boarding a commercial flight and discovered he knew the pilot from the war years. Lamb got off plane, refusing to fly. He had flown with the pilot during the war and thought the man was an unsafe pilot.

Uncle Lamb was known for his bedside manner. It was said that he only had to talk to patients to make them feel better.

My father received a number of gifts from Uncle Lamb during the war and brought some home for him. One of those gifts was a wine bottle from Hitler's wine cellar. It was left at my father's childhood home and someone, not knowing its value or origin, drank it.

IX Troop Carrier Command

North Africa – 1943
Sicily – 1943
Naples-Foggia – 1943-1944
Rome-Anzo – 1944
Normandy – 1944
Central Europe – 1945
Rhineland – 1945

50th Troop Carrier Squadron Stations
Bowman Field, Louisville, Kentucky
January 1942 to November 1943

Sunninghill Park, England
November 1943 to September 1944

Chantilly, France
September 1944 to June 1945

Bad Kissingen, Germany
June 1945 to December 1945

Chapter One
Preparing for Service

"Hey, Doc! Inbound. Causalities," the medical aide yelled as he loped by the tent door. "The pilot radioed. Shots to the fuselage. Three injured. One engine out." Flight surgeon Lamb Myhr snatched up the medical bag he kept supplied for such occasions.

The June 1943 heat in the North African desert hit Lamb like a punch to the face as he pushed through the door. Layers of heat shimmered along the horizon. As Lamb climbed into the jeep, the aide stomped the gas and rocked Lamb back, pressing him into the seat. They sped past the squadron tents dispersed among the rolling sand dunes until they reached the lone flat area the 314th Troop Carrier Group maintained as an airstrip.

A hum grew into a roar as the first of the C-47s came into view. One plane flew outside the standard tight formation, its wing dropping to the right. After that plane, another aircraft also dipped its wing, a small trail of dark smoke billowing out behind it. The plane no longer in formation landed and quickly taxied out of the way. Undamaged planes circled above, letting the injured ones land first.

The smoking airplane touched down, rolled a few yards before its nose hit the runaway, and then skidded sideways. A wing bounced off the ground, bringing the plane to a jerking halt. The right engine burst into flames.

Speeding forward, the aide drove the jeep as close to the plane as possible, arriving just before the ambulance. The heat from the fire drove the already over-one-hundred-degrees desert temperature even higher. The metal skin of the craft ceased rattling as the jeep came to a halt and Lamb jumped out. An asbestos-clad fire crew bounded off a large truck and hustled to smother the flames with foam. Others pushed closer in hopes of saving the flight crew.

"Doc, it's Rogers. He has burns to his hands and feet," a crewman yelled before disappearing into the interior of the plane. A minute later the crewmember reappeared, supporting Rogers with the help of another man. Every crewman worked quickly to carry the injured out onto the wing. The aide handed up a litter. Rogers was placed on the litter and carefully lowered down. Through the haze of black, rolling smoke caught in the unceasing wind, it was difficult to see or breathe.

"Anyone else?" Lamb called.

The flight-crew members shot Lamb a grim look. "Simmons and Rich didn't make it," the crew radio operator told him. His level voice contrasted with the dark emotion reflected in his eyes. "Others are behind me. Mac has a cut. Nothing serious."

"Let's get Rogers on the jeep and away from the plane," Lamb told his aide, and men ran to help. Lamb knew there was a high probability of pilots and co-pilots burning to death during landings, but that knowledge never made the experience any more palpable.

Lamb had no time to worry about what was happening around him. He had a patient to consider and he needed to stabilize Rogers for transport to the hospital.

With the help of the aide, Lamb secured Rogers in the ambulance. "You'll be fine, Rogers. Hang in there," Lamb said as he gave the airman morphine.

Turning to another aide, Lamb ordered, "Check the other man. See that the bleeding is controlled and bring him to the dispensary." Lamb climbed into the ambulance and he and his aide sped away from the burning plane with Rogers.

At the dispensary, Lamb cut away the burned fabric of Roger's flight suit, applied carbolic acid and phenol, and covered it with gauze impregnated with Vaseline, which worked like a local anesthetic over the red, angry skin. It was a slow but effective process. This method of burn care helped relieve pain and hyperemia and had recently become standard procedure.

Rogers moaned. Lamb waved his hand over Rogers to

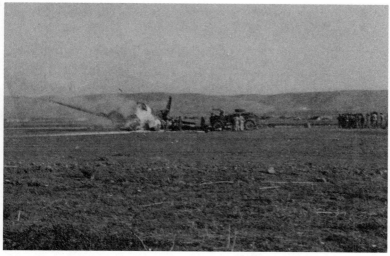

C-47 crash, Africa

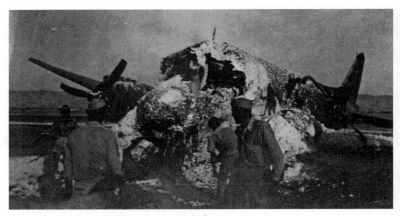

Fire of a crashed C-47 put out with foam

keep the flies at bay. "We'll get you on a plane and out of here as soon as possible."

Crashed, burning planes were a regular occurrence and a risk of flying for the aircrews of the United States Army Air Forces during World War II. Scenes like this one would occur numerous times before the twenty-five-year-old doctor returned to Tennessee at the war's end.

Flight surgeon Lamb Bolton Myhr was born May 8, 1917, in Bellevue, Tennessee, just outside of Nashville. His father was twenty-two years older than his mother and nearly sixty years old when Lamb joined the family. The fifth and last child of a Christian Church minister from Norway and a college-educated Latin teacher from East Tennessee, Lamb had three sisters and one brother.

Provided with an excellent education, Lamb attended Davidson County Schools and later went to Tate Boarding School in Shelbyville, Tennessee, until it closed. He returned to Nashville to complete high school at Duncan Preparatory School. He later graduated from Vanderbilt University with a bachelor of arts degree. One of his professors was so impressed with Lamb's excellent memory that the professor encouraged him to attend medical school. In 1935, one applicant out of nine was selected to attend the Vanderbilt University School of Medicine, an institution that ranked third behind Harvard and Johns Hopkins as the best medical school in the nation. Lamb took his professor's advice and applied; he entered Vanderbilt medical school in the fall of 1936.

His first year of medical study consisted of classes in gross anatomy, histology, neurology, bio-chemistry, and physiology. Anatomy was Lamb's most difficult subject, and he complained that the smell of formaldehyde stayed with him no matter what he did to try to remove it.

The total cost of the first year of medical school at Vanderbilt was $743.40, which included $125.00 for a required microscope. The US surgeon general stepped up training in medical schools because of the fear of impending war. Lamb's schooling was paid for through a government assistance program, the goal of which was to train as many doctors as possible in preparation for war. Nine-month-long classes were instituted with almost no free time between terms. Students attended medical school year-round under the 9-9-9 Program, which allowed two classes to be training at the same time by accelerating the time necessary to complete the program. Medical students spent two nine-month periods doing premedical training, four nine-month periods of medical training, and then completed a nine-month internship.

The second year included classes in bacteriology, pathology, pharmacology, physical diagnosis, clinical pathology, and parasitic diseases. Case studies and grand rounds filled the rest of the first two years. Medicine, surgery, surgical pathology, and obstetrics composed the third year. In 1938, clinical students at Vanderbilt medical school were obligated to see patients in addition to doing lab work, and they were also required to deliver at least five babies in the home.

Lamb's fourth and final year included medicine, surgery, preventive medicine, public health pediatrics, and gynecology classes. Hours of hands-on training were gained working at Thayer-Harding VA Hospital in Nashville. There was a three-month rotation in each of the areas of surgery, medicine, emergency, and obstetrics and gynecology.

World events were encroaching on the young doctor's education. Great Britain was already at war with Germany, and during Lamb's medical school years there were a number of guest lecturers from Europe. The 1940-41 school catalogue stated that Sir Edward Mellanby, director of the Medical Research Council of Great Britain, was on the agenda. The catalogue also included a disclaimer from the committee that invited guest speakers stating that they hoped circumstances in Europe would not prevent Sir Mellanby from visiting Nashville.

Lamb spent the summer of 1940 working with the Cocke County Department of Public Health in Newport, Tennessee, caring for the people who lived in that mountainous region. He graduated from medical school in the spring of 1941. Fifty people made up the new group of doctors: forty-nine men and one woman. Lamb and five of his fellow graduates were classmates through Duncan Preparatory High

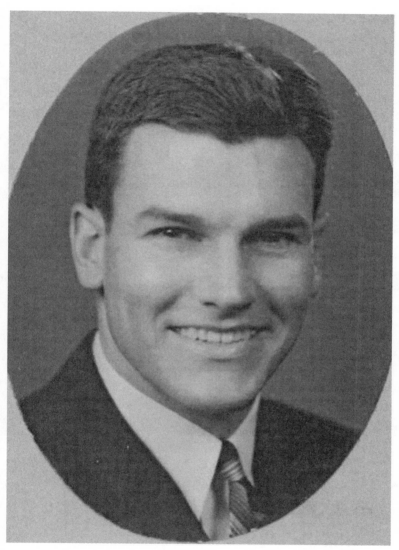

Lamb's portrait in the Vanderbilt University School of Medicine Class of 1941 photo (Courtesy Historical Collection, Eskind Biomedical Library, Vanderbilt University Medical Center)

School, Vanderbilt undergraduate, and Vanderbilt medical school. They would later see each other during the war.

With "MD" behind his name and a plan to specialize in internal medicine, Lamb moved to Birmingham, Alabama, to do his one year of residency at Hillman-Jefferson Hospital. There residents dressed in all white and earned ten dollars a day. One of Lamb's older sisters and her family lived in Birmingham, which made it nice to be assigned to that internship.

On December 8, 1941, Lamb had only been in Birmingham for a few months when he woke to the radio report that the Japanese had bombed Pearl Harbor. The next day, President Roosevelt declared war on Germany and Japan. Like most American men, the young doctor wanted to join the military right away.

Lamb's medical superiors advised him to wait six months before enlisting so he could complete his medical training and qualify as medical personnel. Their advice paid off as doctors would be desperately needed in the years ahead. Lamb finished his residency in March of 1942. Around the same time, after several long months of waiting, he enlisted, though he would have soon been drafted if he had not voluntarily signed up.

All of Lamb's medical school classmates joined the military with the exception of the lone female student. While still in Birmingham, Lamb wrote home to say that he had heard from the Medical Army Air Corps. He would probably report on July 1. He hoped to travel to Maxwell Field in Montgomery, Alabama, to see if he might be stationed there. He thought the war was at a turning point and would not last another year.

Lamb would later write that he believed he would be sent to Carlisle, Pennsylvania. He planned to buy his uniform before he went into the service. The cost of a uniform would be $150; he wanted to purchase the uniform in Birmingham because he thought he could get a better quality one than he would find on a post. He also thought he might get to work in a defense plant while waiting to be called up.

On May 16, 1942, the five-foot-ten, dark-haired man with smooth, Scandinavian skin, easy smile, and gentle laugh married Betty Freeland of Nashville. They honeymooned in Highlands, North Carolina. Betty had three brothers who were already serving in the military.

Lamb's father had died while Lamb was in high school. Before his marriage, Lamb lived in a house primarily filled with females. His mother, his oldest unmarried sister, and his next-to-oldest widowed sister and her young son all lived there. Naturally, questions about whom Lamb was dating were frequent. Whenever they were posed, Lamb pithily responded by telling them with a grin that he was seeing "Lucy Fullbosom." This private man was almost married to Betty before the family knew he was dating her.

Lamb received his call up in June 1942. He was stationed in Nashville, where one of three Flying Training Command classification centers was located. (The others were in San Antonio, Texas, and Santa Ana, California.) In Nashville, Lamb went through a six-week practical training course. Part of his time was devoted to the medical processing of men, and the other part was used to familiarize him with medical administration and the unique issues of aviation medicine.

Lamb had become a member of the Army Air Forces, which had changed from the Army Air Corps in 1941. The Army Air Forces provided doctors, nurses, flight surgeons, and corpsmen. These men would be responsible for setting up field hospitals and battalion aid stations. Lamb requested assignment as a flight surgeon.

Thousands of dedicated medical practitioners volunteered for aviation medical responsibilities that were often undefined or unfamiliar to them. Very few flight surgeons trained as actual surgeons in medical school; most studied to be primary-care physicians.

The term "flight surgeon" comes from an era when all military physicians were referred to as surgeons. To qualify as a flight surgeon, an individual had to graduate from a Class A medical school, complete one year of a rotating internship, and complete a month-long course at the School of Aviation Medicine. These doctors were responsible for the medical treatment and certification of aviation personnel, which included pilots and aircrew. Public-health and preventative-medicine concerns also fell to the flight surgeon. In addition to dispensing routine medical services and managing traumatic injury cases, flight surgeons selected men for flight training, putting an emphasis on the ophthalmological, cardiovascular, and neuropsychiatric qualifications of the men. They were also to study the effects of flight on an aircrew, serve as confidante and advisor to the men, and be their intermediary with the commanding officer. There were three components to the military medical organization: physical examinations, field medical services (which handled battle casualties), and hospitals.

As a 1st lieutenant in the Medical Corps, Lamb spent the fall of 1942 at Randolph Field, Texas, at the School of Aviation Medicine. Betty stayed behind in Tennessee. Lamb enjoyed the day-long classes and found them instructive, believing they would be helpful when applied practically.

From late August 1940 to the end of the war, about four thousand doctors entered and completed the basic aviation medical examiner program. Approximately half of those satisfied further learning and experience requirements to qualify as full-fledged certified flight surgeons by taking classes through the School of Aviation Medicine. The additional classes included nutrition, physical fitness, mental stress of flying, and the need for convalescence. A class on aviation physiology was required for all flight surgeons. Additionally, information was provided on chemical warfare.

Lamb completed the program and became a certified flight surgeon, earning a Flight Surgeon Badge as a commissioned medical officer. He also wore Flight Surgeon Wings. This pin looked much like a pilot's, but it was gold rather than silver and featured a caduceus in the center.

After aviation school, Lamb was stationed at Bowman Field in Louisville, Kentucky, as part of the 349th Evacuation Unit of the Ninth Air Force. When Lamb and his wife, Betty, arrived at Bowman Field, they were housed for a time at the Brown Hotel in downtown Louisville. They later settled at a tourist travel court, Sunset Lodge, about five miles from the Field. Also staying in the same lodge were six other doctors

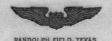

RANDOLPH FIELD, TEXAS

School of Aviation Medicine,
September 27, 1942.

Dearest Mother,

Sorry you haven't heard from me before this, but a card I mailed to you Monday was returned today for postage.

I am enjoying this course very much. It is extremely informative and well-organized. The instructors are well-trained men. This has been an extremely fortunate break for me. I was informed that I am the youngest person (doctor) to attend this school in 10-12 years. I am unable to say when I shall leave here.

The President was here today.

Hope you are well and give my regards to all the family.

Love,

Lamb Britton.

Letter written from Randolph Field by Lamb to his mother, 1942

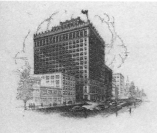

The Brown Hotel

BROADWAY AT FOURTH AVE.

HAROLD E. HARTER
MANAGER

Louisville   Kentucky

Saturday

Dear Mrs. Taylor –

Well here we are semi-settled in a tourist court. Most of the officers from Nashville all arrived at about the same time Thursday and after having dinner together we all stayed at the above Hotel. For a well advertised place the Brown Hotel is certainly the worst we've ever seen. All our rooms were perfectly filthy. There were bottles, cigarettes, papers, dirty linen strewn everywhere but even with all that we were lucky to get a room at all. By virtue of comparison this little tourist court is heaven. It is out about seven miles from town and our twelve miles from Bowman Field. We are lucky in as much as there are six doctors and their wives staying here and five cars so that the gas rationing and transportation will be no problem. The men plan to go together to the Field and get their breakfast on the way. I got special permission to use my coffee and toast electrical gadgets and two of us wives have coffee and toast or we could walk down the

Letter from the Brown Hotel, Louisville, Kentucky

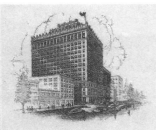

The
Brown Hotel
BROADWAY AT FOURTH AVE.

HAROLD E. HARTER
MANAGER

Louisville   Kentucky

highway to several joints for breakfast
and lunch. Neither of us are particularly
anxious to go out for three meals a day
so we plan to get along on a little
fruit and whatever we can keep in
our rooms. At night we all drive
over to the little town of Shively for
our evening meal — it's only about a
mile from here and there's a little café
there which serves very good home-cooked
meals.

Our room is quite large, bright, and
cheerful and done up in very nice taste
and rather good furniture. We are
really pleased with it.

We know no more about how long
we'll be here than we did when we
left Nashville. Three of the men have
already been sent out and the rest (a
total of 23 doctors) told to be ready
to leave anytime on a 12-24-48 hour
notice. The whole idea of air-transport
evacuation is so new that no one
can guess how long it will take
to become organized.

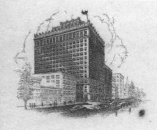

The
Brown Hotel
BROADWAY AT FOURTH AVE.

HAROLD E. HARTER
MANAGER

Louisville   Kentucky

we are saving the fruit-cake for
Christmas but it will be hard waiting.
I know it must be delicious and it
will be awfully nice to have such
a nice little bit of home in our new
surroundings.

Lamb is positively itching to know
what's in Eline's package but he will
just have to itch until Dec. 25th.

Please tell Ivan Sue how proud I
am of the dainty little knit things. I
know how much time and effort must
have gone into the making of them – and
I truly do appreciate her thoughtfulness.
Give every one our love and best
wishes for a merry Christmas.
                Much love,
                    Betty and Lamb

c/o Sunset Lodge - No. 12
    Shively, Kentucky

and their wives. There were five cars between the couples, and they often ate their evening meals out together at a local café. Lamb and Betty's room was nothing more than a small hotel room. Lamb spent his days on the air base while Betty awaited his return. In the mornings, they shared a small breakfast in their room prepared over a one-eye hot plate.

Bowman Field opened in November 1942 for flight training. The base housed combat-readiness training schools and glider-pilot-combat training schools and was designated as the Army Air Force School to train flight surgeons, medical techs, and flight nurses. Bowman Field was located five miles from downtown Louisville and was the busiest field in the country. The construction of barracks, mess halls, and other facilities to meet needs of the overwhelming number of people stationed at the field cost a million dollars.

The graduates of the school would evaluate and treat half a million sick and wounded airmen before the end of the war. Medical personnel who attended the school learned to treat and evacuate wounded by air, while acquiring skills to help ensure survival in combat zones.

The training at Bowman for glider pilots was less about flying and more about military training with weapons and procedures for what to do on the ground. The men learned to use a rifle, fire hand guns, and throw grenades. They were also trained in patrol techniques, scouting, compass use, and map reading. They participated in close and extend drills, forced cross-country marches, night bivouacs, tactical formations, chemical warfare, infantry organization, combat swimming, and military courtesy.

Pilots came from almost all walks of life—rich, poor,

cities, and farms. Many had attended college, and the majority had finished high school, which was unusual for a man of the 1930s. Pilots tended to be white Anglo-Saxon Protestants.

Batteries of tests were established to determine if a man would make a good member of a flight crew, particularly a pilot. These tests differed from year to year. Most of the psychological tests turned out to be unsuccessful or inadequate in making a determination and were scrapped. In 1941, aptitude tests were devised that would indicate the applicant's general potentialities, practical judgment, and ability to take instruction. Further tests were given to measure a man's aptitude to be a pilot, bomber, or navigator. By 1942, the Air Surgeon Office reinstated the neuropsychiatric examination, believing the attitude and aptitude tests did not clearly define a man's ability to perform.

A pilot's physical examination was lengthy. It included everything from recording basic information, like height and weight, to an extensive eye exam requiring numerous eye charts and tests to rule out heart disease. It was necessary to file a different form for each exam. Psychological questions were also asked; there were more than fifty of them, covering everything from a man's family life to health history.

In the specialty of aviation medicine, five areas were considered to determine if an applicant was fit to become a flyer. The first was his physical condition, or how he reacted to the loss of oxygen in the blood at extreme heights and how he adjusted to the cold. The second was his reaction to gravitational pull. This dealt with the speed and maneuvers made in a plane during flights. Third was

PHYSICAL EXAMINATION FOR FLYING
(See AR 40-100, 40-105, 40-110)

201

COLORED

1. _____ (MI) Aviation Cadet-Pilot 14069047 25 5/12
(Last name) (First name) (Middle initial) (Grade and arm or service) (Serial No.) (Age) (Years service)

2. TAAF., Tuskegee, Alabama For Appointment & Extended Active Duty Jan. 1943 Qualified
(Address) (Purpose of examination) (Date and result last examination)

_____ Flying time as: Pilot 141.2 ; observer ___ ; pilot ___ ; observer ___
(Aeronautical rating) (Total) (Total) (Last 6 mos.) (Last 6 mos.)

3. Temperature 98.6 Vaccinations: Typhoid series, No. 1 Last 1-27-43; smallpox 2-13-43 Reaction Vaccinia
(Date)

4. Medical history.
(In the case of applicant include family. Has he ever had epilepsy, enuresis, headaches, dizziness, vertigo, fainting, stammering, tic, somnambulism, pavor nocturnus, nightmares, rheumatic diseases, anxiety trends, irritability, apathy, elation, depression, sensory disturbances, enuresis, asthma, unconsciousness, repeated episodes of alcoholism, complicated pneumonia, syphilis, renal calculi, tuberculosis, asthma, hay fever, repeated colds, mastoiditis, sinusitis, tonsillitis, arthritis in any form, malaria, severe injuries, major operations, or other pertinent history? Explain fully.)

Usual childhood diseases. Family history negative. Denies any operations, injuries
or serious illness.

_____

_____

_____

5. Eye: Inspection Normal   Nystagmus None
6. Associated parallel movements Normal   Pupils: Equality Equal   Reaction Normal
7. Visual acuity: R. E. 20/20 ___, correctible to 20/ ___ L. E. 20/20 ___, correctible to 20/ ___
8. Depth perception (uncorrected) 6 ___ mm. With correction ___ mm.
9. Heterophoria at 6 meters: Eso 0 ___ Exo 0 ___ R. H. 0 ___ L. H. 0 ___ Prism divergence 8 ___
10. Red lens test Normal   Angle convergence: PcB 66 mm. Pd 62 mm. 51 °
11. Accommodation: R. 10 ___ D. L. 10 ___ D. Addition required for 50 cm. R. ___ L. ___
(Jaeger type): Right J. -1-18 ___, correctible to J. ___ ; Left J-1-18 ___, correctible to J. ___
12. Color vision Passes A.O.C. book
13. Field of vision (form): R. Normal ___ L. Normal ___ Ophthalmoscopic: R. Normal ___ L. Normal ___
14. Refraction: R. reads 20/20 with Not Required CAx ° L. reads 20/20 with Not Required CAx °
15. Ear: History of ear trouble Denies
16. External ear: R. Normal ___ L. Normal ___ Membrana tympani: R. Normal ___ L. Normal ___
17. Hearing (whisper): R. 20/20. L. 20/20. Audiometer (percent loss): R. ___ L. ___
18. Nares Normal   Tonsils Present NS-ND
19. Teeth:
    (a)   Right   (Examiner's)   Left
        8 7 X 5 4 3 2 1   1 2 3 4 5 6 7 8   Indicate: Restorable carious teeth by O; nonrestorable carious teeth by /;
       16 15 X 13 12 11 10 9   9 10 11 12 13 X 15 X   missing natural teeth by X.
    (b) Remarks, including other defects None
    (c) Prosthetic appliances None   (d) Classification IV
20. History of swing, train, air, or sea sickness Denies
21. Barany chair (when indicated with results) Not indicated
22. Posture Good   Figure Medium   Frame Medium
        (Erectest, good, fair, bad)   (slender, medium, stocky, obese)   (Light, medium, heavy)
23. Height 74 inches. Weight 135 pounds. Chest: Inspiration 39 ; Expiration 35 Rest 36 Abdomen 31
24. Skin and lymphatics Normal   Endocrine system Normal
25. Bones, joints, muscles Normal
                                                 Feet Pes Planus 2°bil. NS-ND
26. Heart Normal
27. Pulse rate, 55-75 . B.P.: S110-120 . D. 70-80 . Schneider /15 . Pulse immediately after exercise 95
    Two minutes after exercise 75 . Character Full & regular
28. Arteries Normal   Varicose veins None

[Regimental appointment as cadet, examination in the Air Corps, examination in Air Corps Reserve, transfer to the Air Corps, or any other special purpose. 10-23191]
[I, II, III, or IV; see par. 5, AR 40-110.]

W. D., A. G. O., Form No. 64
(May 22, 1941)

Physical examination form used by flight surgeons, page one (Courtesy the Air Force Historical Research Agency)

202

29. Respiratory system Normal
30. X-ray of chest [1] Negative
31. Abdominal viscera Normal
32. Hernia None   Hemorrhoids None
33. Genito-urinary system Normal
34. Nervous system: Reflexes, gait, coordination, musculature, tension, tremor, and other pertinent tests
     Normal
35. Laboratory procedures: Kahn [1] Negative   Wassermann [1]
     Urinalysis: Reaction Acid Sp. gr. 1.018 Albumin Negative Sugar Negative Microscopical Negative
36. Estimated adaptability for military aeronautics (if unsatisfactory, state reasons)
     Satisfactory

37. Remarks on conditions not sufficiently described Examinee states he is not drawing a pension,
     disability allowance, compensation or retired pay from the U.S. Government.

38. Is the examinee physically qualified for flying duty? Yes If yes, in what class? 1
     If disqualified, indicate defects by paragraph number —
39. Have defects been waived by The Adjutant General? — If yes, give date —
     If no, is waiver recommended? — Is request for waiver attached? —
40. Is the examinee incapacitated for active service? No If yes, indicate defect by paragraph number —
41. Corrective measures or other action recommended —

42. If applicant for appointment: Does he meet physical requirements? Yes Do you recommend acceptance with minor
     physical defects? — If rejection is recommended, specify cause —

Station Hospital,
Tuskegee Army Air Field,
Tuskegee, Alabama   June 21, 1943   RICHARD C. CUMMING, Lt. Col.   Medical Corps.
     (Place)   (Date)   (Name and grade)

                                          HAROLD E. THORNELL, Major,   Medical Corps.
                                          (Name and grade)
REVIEWED AND APPROVED:
RICHARD C. CUMMING, Lt./ Col., Medical Corps.   E. BROWN SINGLETON, Captain,   Medical Corps.
     (Senior flight surgeon)   (Name and grade)

                              1st Ind.[2]

Headquarters _____ 19___
To the Commanding General _____
     Remarks and recommendations _____

_____
                              (Grade)   (organization and arm or service)
                                                              Commanding.

                              2d Ind.[3]
_____ 19___ To The Adjutant General.
_____

[1] Required for candidates for commission, Reserve officers reporting for extended active duty, and applicants for flying cadet.
[2] State action taken on recommendation of the board. If incapacitated for active service, state whether action by retiring board is recommended.
NOTE.—Use typewriter if practicable. Attach additional plate sheets if required.

Physical examination form used by flight surgeons, page two (Courtesy
the Air Force Historical Research Agency)

psychological issues, which included how a man reacted in a crisis and how well he dealt with stress. The fourth was physiological, having to do with how the man oriented or failed to orient himself during flight, including his depth perception, reaction time, and ability to tolerate motion that might confuse him. The last was his emotional level. Doctors looked for the man with strong emotional currents who gained a gratification and importance from flying, which in turn seemed to shield him from thoughts of failure or death.

Medical standards for entry into the military were lowered after war was declared. Men in good physical condition were difficult to find, as many lived with poor nutrition and little or no medical care during the Depression. Finding men best suited to flight was paramount. The ideal pilot was a graduate of a military academy who became a flyer, was in near to perfect physical condition, and was emotionally, physiologically, and psychologically sound.

The workload to determine who would make flight crews grew by the thousands for flight surgeons after war was declared. Air Force commanders were uncompromising in their need for air personnel, as were the Army and Navy. Prior to 1939, the rejection rate for flyers was 73.2 percent, and after realistic downgrades the rejection rate went to 50.3 percent. The majority of the men rejected for pilot status were reclassified as air crewmen to become bombardiers, navigators, or fight engineers. The decision not to lower the intellectual and physical standards for aviation cadets was never seriously challenged. It became evident that the complexities of modern aircraft and the nature of aerial warfare demanded pilots and crew be chosen from the best of the best, based on both physical and mental standards.

The Standard Form 64 was the official guideline used to assess each crewmember. This special report dealt with the physical and psychological status of a pilot, used to evaluate the flying officer's capabilities for carrying out necessary special duties. It was regularly filled out on each flying officer in the squadron to determine whether the man was "medically fit to fly."

Military airplanes were flying faster and higher than ever before, creating new medical issues. Determining why 90 percent of pilots became disoriented enough to crash planes became a high priority. Flight surgeons also studied other factors having to do with flight.

The five main medical risks during World War II concerning a pilot were anoxia, frostbite, aero-otitis, battle wounds, and stress. Anoxia is critical lack of oxygen from flying at a high attitude. It can cause a man to be cyanotic, to have shallow breathing and a weak pulse, or to lose consciousness, the result of which was too often the loss of planes and men. Anoxia was studied to improve flying conditions, and recommendations were made for treatment (pure oxygen).

In 1943, the emphasis turned to teaching airmen how to survive at high altitudes and how to prevent illness or death from anoxia. The resulting prevention program contributed to a major drop in the accident rate and an almost-as-significant drop in the death rate of crewmen. Gen. Henry Harley "Hap" Arnold, commander of the US Army Air Force, ordered all flight surgeons to fly regularly in order to better understand the aviation environment, study the effects flying had on the crew, and learn the procedures pilots and crewmembers were required to follow. Flight surgeons were considered aircrew members, and to qualify for flight pay they had to fly four hours a month. They also received instruction in conduct while in an airplane, which included bail-out procedures and the use of a parachute.

The second concern was frostbite, caused by sustained temperatures between zero and ten degrees Fahrenheit. Having enough protective equipment available and using it properly was a continuing issue.

Aero-otitis is an acute or chronic middle-ear disorder that often afflicted pilots, causing pain or, even worse, deafness. This type of ear trouble is created when the fluid in the ear does not adjust during high-altitude flights. Later, the pilots often developed an infection.

The fourth concern was battle casualties, which occur naturally during war and were as much a mental as a physical problem. From missing buddies in the next bunk to thinking his number would be the next to come up, each man was forced to face death's clout.

Stress, the fifth of the main concerns, went hand in hand with the fourth. The stress of successfully completing missions, winning the war, living in ugly conditions, being away from home, and so much more had to be addressed by Lamb.

In his "care of the flyer," Lamb attended to six functional areas of each man's health: 1) he evaluated the influence of illness and injury of the man's ability to fly and provided treatment; 2) he treated injuries and disorders caused by flying; 3) he received altitude training and became proficient in the use of oxygen equipment; 4) he taught and evaluated the man's use of protective devices; 5) he diagnosed emotional issues; and 6) he helped the airmen recognize and deal with tension and anxiety. The last two were the most difficult for flight surgeons to successfully discharge.

With Lamb's help, pilots left Bowman Field in top physical condition, mentally alert and confident they could successfully carry out any assigned mission. All the medical training and experience Lamb gained while at Bowman would become invaluable when he went overseas.

While at Bowman Field Betty wrote home: "We know no more about how long we'll be here than we did when we left Nashville. Three of the men have already been sent out and the rest (a total of 23 doctors) told to be ready to leave anytime on a 12-24-48 hour notice. The whole idea of air-transport evacuation is so new that no one can guess how long it will take to become organized."

Lamb's orders came in January 1943, when he was sent to Sedalia AAB, Warrensburg, Missouri, as flight surgeon for the 341th. The then-pregnant Betty traveled with him. He was responsible for the care of three hundred men. On February 26, not long after the move, Lamb returned from leave to receive the news he had been made captain. He would now be making $393 per month.

Capt. Lamb B. Myhr, USAAF, MC (United States Army Air Force, Medical Corps Flight Surgeon), was then assigned to the Ninth Army Air Force, IX Troop Carrier Command (TCC), 52nd Troop Carrier Wing (TCW), 314th Troop Carrier Group (TCG), 50th Troop Carrier Squadron

(TCS). The 50th was one of four squadrons that comprised the 314th TCG. Completing the group were the 32nd, 61st, and the 62nd Troop Carrier Squadrons. Twelve to fourteen planes comprised a squadron, which included all the necessary personnel.

In March, Betty returned to Nashville to prepare for the birth of their child. That month, Lamb would spend time at Fort Bragg, Pope Field, and Laurinburg-Maxton AAB, all in North Carolina. April 1943 was spent at Lawson Field in Georgia, but Lamb did manage to make it home for the birth of his first son in mid-April.

The Ninth Air Force was originally constituted in England in 1941 as the 5 Air Support Command and activated later in 1941 as an airborne and transport operation. It was redesigned as the 9 Air Force in April 1942. After pulling men from other forces, the 9 Air Force was reconstituted as the Ninth Air Force in September 1942. The bomber command of the Ninth Air Force moved to North Africa in November of 1942.

Part of the Ninth Air Force, the IX Troop Carrier Command (IX TCC) was composed of light and medium bombers, two fighter commands, and a troop carrier command. Each command consisted of a number of wings, usually three. Wings were comprised of three or four groups, and they in turn contained three squadrons of bombers and fighters and four squadrons of troop carriers each. The IX TCC trained in Sedalia, Missouri, and Lawson Field in Georgia.

Lamb was responsible for the medical care of around five hundred men who were assigned to the 314th Troop Carrier Group, including crewmen, mechanics, and supply personnel. He and the two male aides assigned to him were three out of the ten men necessary behind the front line to support one fighting man. In *Green Light! A Troop Carrier Squadron's War From Normandy to the Rhine*, Martin Wolfe writes: "our airplane pilots and their abilities were the main reason the rest of us were also there. Pilots, however, were only the cutting edge of a large and complex operation. They amounted to fewer than one-tenth the total squadron roster—forty out of about 420, when we were at maximum strength in Europe. We also needed navigators, glider pilots, crew chiefs, and radio operators, communications experts, cooks, supply managers, sheet-metal men (for repairing holes in a plane's skin), dope and fabric men (for repairing holes in gliders), and several other sorts of technicians."[1]

Lamb began making preparations for his deployment to North Africa. He was issued the standard field equipment for overseas service in a combat unit, which consisted of flying equipment, a bedroll, gas mask, and pistol. Officers in tactical units were also issued a belt, cap, service jacket, underwear and undershirts (cotton and wool), gloves (dress white, leather, and woolen), six handkerchiefs, lace shoes, black tie, overcoat, overshoes, rubber raincoat, flannel shirts, brown shoes, six pair of socks, officer's belt, comb, footlocker, razor, soap, and two towels.

Lamb was allowed forty pounds of baggage, including his coat and anything he might be carrying in his pockets. The flight bag issued by the Army was the only baggage permitted. Small items packed for deployment included extra razor blades, matches, lighter fluid and flints, chocolate bars, flashlight batteries, extra insignia, and essential jewelry.

Benefitting from the knowledge of those with previous

military experience in the area, Lamb packed tooth powder, which worked better than toothpaste in the desert, and a shaving stick, which yielded more shaves than shaving soap. It was recommended that officers carry $400 in a money belt for emergencies, in case they needed to pay for food and shelter. Lamb normally dressed in coveralls or the pants/shirt combination doctors were issued. Officers wore boots under their slacks instead of shoes.

In preparation for his deployment, Lamb received his shots, collected his dog tags, saw to his insurance, checked and rechecked his equipment, filled out a notice of address change, received a physical, listened to lectures on security, reviewed the packing list, packed and repacked, and was instructed to write out a will. He designated Betty as beneficiary of his $10,000 National Service Life Insurance policy.

With a great deal of angst and concern, Lamb left his wife and his two-and-a-half-week-old baby boy. Betty and their son would live in a small house that she and Lamb had purchased in Nashville just after they married. Lamb's small family would await his return there.

The young doctor's transport to the front was a lengthy one. He departed Morrison Field in West Palm Beach, Florida, on May 6, 1943, in a C-47 (plane number 42-23402), and arrived in Puerto Rico the same day. On May 8, his plane flew a search mission around St. Lucia. Bad weather kept them grounded for a number of days.

On May 13, Lamb wrote his family that he had the most enjoyable time on a beautiful tropical island in the British West Indies. It was a wonderful place, with a constant

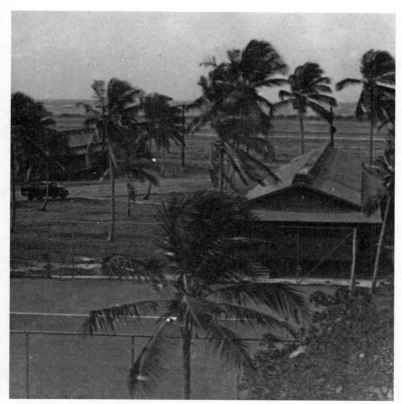

Saint Lucia, British West Indies

breeze off the ocean, and quite cool. He spent time picking bananas, coconuts, pineapples, and orchids and also visited a leper colony, one of the oldest in the world.

Late in the day on May 14, Lamb arrived at Atkinson Field, Trinidad, to fly the next day to Belem, Brazil, after which he would fly to Natel, Brazil. On May 17 the plane flew to Ascension Island in the middle of the South Atlantic. It was considered a feat of navigation to find islands in the

Atlantic Ocean. The plane stayed there a day so the crew could rest. On May 19 Lamb arrived in Dakar, West Africa, and flew on to Marrakech, Morocco, for refueling before reaching his final destination of Berguent, Morocco, thirteen days after leaving the United States.

The 50th War Diary, the official record of the 50th Troop Carrier Squadron, for June 1943 to August 1943 reads as follows:

> The Air echelon, under the command of Captain Joseph H. McClure, with thirteen C-47's and personnel of thirty-seven officers and forty-eight enlisted men, left Lawson Field, Fort Benning, Georgia, on the fifth day of May for Morrison Field, West Palm Beach, Florida, where it was staged, departing thence on the seventh of May for its base in Africa by way of Borinquen, Porto Rico [sic]; Saint Lucia, British West Indies; Atkinson Field, Georgetown, British Guinea; Belen, Brazil; Natal Ascension Islands, Dakar, Africa; Marrakech, French Morocco; and Oujda. The air echelon arrived at Berguent Army Air Field [sic] on the twenty-first day of May, 1943.[2]

William Randolph Hearst, who became a print-media mogul after the war, piloted the plane that transported Lamb to Africa.

Chapter Two
North Africa

In November 1942, American and British troops made their first joint amphibious invasion. Known as Operation Torch, it was a successful movement into North Africa. By December, German Field Marshal Erwin Rommel had retreated to a strong fortification near the Mareth Line, which huddled all the Axis forces within the border of Tunisia. The Mareth Line, built by the French before WWII, had been used to stop invasions from Libya. This line was the Germans' last point of defense in southern Tunisia.

By February 1943, the Allies controlled the waters of the Mediterranean. German supply lines had been safe prior to this date because the distance between Allied airfields in Egypt and those supply lines was too great; but with the Allies now so close to the coast, the situation had changed.

The Ninth Air Force left the Egyptian delta and moved to the Gambut area in February 1943, ending the long return flight to Egypt for refueling. Headquarters was established in El-Adem. In March 1943, the Allied forces moved on to Algeria to the El-Assa landing ground. This stationed planes eighty miles from the front and twenty miles from the sea. From this location, the Mediterranean was controlled by air and the Air Force was in a position to bomb Naples, Italy, bringing about the defeat of the Mareth Line. On Palm

AFRICA

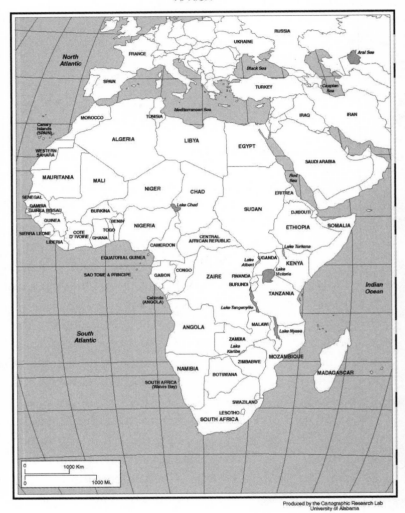

Sunday, April 1943, after a major bombing of the transport area of Tunis, the Axis troops in North Africa were defeated.

Lt. Gen. Ira Eaker commanded the Mediterranean Allied Air Force. The theater covered the entire Mediterranean from Casablanca, Morocco, on the Atlantic to Curio, Egypt, at the edge of Asia. The force was gigantic and composed of predominantly American planes and pilots with some British and a few French personnel.

From the air station in Benghazi, Libya, the Ninth Air Force could attack fighter production in southern Germany and Austria 1,200 miles away. The Allied Air Force could also reach and bomb Ploesti, Romania, from this position; as the site of a vast complex of crude oil refineries that supplied Germany with thirty-five percent of its oil, Ploesti was a valuable target for the Allies.

Lamb arrived in Africa in late May 1943. He exchanged his pristine white medical uniform for the tan desert uniform and heavy boots of the Army Air Force. The cool green hills of Tennessee were a distant memory in the stifling heat of the Sahara Desert.

He reported to Maj. Quinn M. Corley, who commanded both the pilots and paratroopers at the Liege/ Bierset, Morocco, field known as Field A-93. Fields were given letters and numbers as names because it was often difficult to identify them by geographic location. Field A-93 was little more than a flat spot in the middle of an arid valley. Lamb served as adviser to Major Corley in "all areas of fitness." As flight surgeon, Lamb's concern would be with not only the individual pilot but also the aircrew of multi-engine planes and the men as a team.

EUROPE

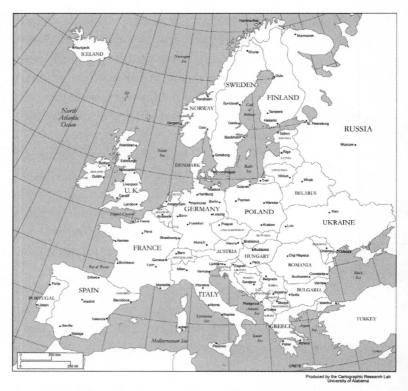

Produced by the Cartographic Research Lab
University of Alabama

From Africa, the Ninth Air Force could target strategic areas in Europe, particularly Italy, Germany, Austria, and Romania

Morocco—or, in the words of 50th TCS pilot Gordon D. Binghan, the "land of sand and sweat"—was a country of scalding hot days and freezing nights. The normal temperature could soar beyond one hundred degrees, and there was no relief in the form of rain. "The heat was oppressive and unrelenting," a crewman wrote. The new men arriving were met by those already there and told how

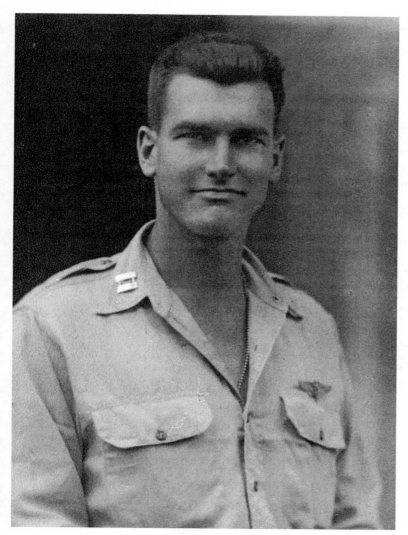

Capt. Lamb B. Myhr in North Africa, 1943

rough living conditions were. The residents pointed the men to their housing, tents across the field barely visible through the dust and heat waves generated by the desert.

Cacti grew everywhere. It was hot inside the square and pyramidal tents, and the airplanes and vehicles were hot to the touch. Summer days could be so scorching that water left in jerry-cans heated to the point where a person would be burned if he tried to touch it. The lucky men were stationed near the shelter of an olive grove.

Every couple of weeks, water for drinking and bathing was trucked into camp. The men looked forward to the trucks' arrival and had to be quick to get a bath once they made a delivery; often there was not enough water for everyone. Showers were rare and highly anticipated. Then men quickly squirted themselves to get wet and soap up and then rinsed off with another quick squirt. The walk in high temperatures to get back to the living quarters meant the men needed another bath by the time they arrived at the tents. Portable bags known as Lyster bags were used to supply troops with purified drinking water.

Sirocco, a continuous wind from the south, could blow twenty-four hours a day over the northern Mediterranean coast for months without ceasing. Flying sand was an ongoing problem year-round, but it was particularly dangerous during the Sirocco season. This hot, dry wind that came off the Sahara Desert generated dust and often created sand storms that grounded planes. Poor visibility was a constant problem and made living conditions intolerable. Special care was taken to keep the sand off the wounded's injuries, but many times it was impossible to avoid.

Sand was not only a concern for medical reasons but also

because it often caused maintenance issues in equipment, particularly instruments. The dirt was particularly hard on the cooling systems of the planes and caused the engines to cut out. It was not unusual to make fifty engine changes in one plane due to grit. Replacing a plane's engine was not a simple task; the process required at least nine men per engine to ensure proper removal and refit.

For hundreds of miles, the land surrounding Lamb was nothing more than monochromatic shades of beige. Even the buildings in the small villages and few, scattered inland towns were the same dirty light brown. This description of an Army Air Force camp established in North Africa was given by Maj. John R. Kane in his diary: "The building area of the camp is to the east of the highway, and is shaded from the afternoon sun by the tall eucalyptus trees that line both sides of the road. The camp was erected in an olive grove with each building so placed that a minimum of trees were disturbed. The result is a pleasing dispersal of the camp among the olive trees." Kane continues with a description of the camp's structures, which were "made of native stone and roofed with sheet iron. There will be enough housing for two squadrons to provide for all the men and officers, and in addition have space for offices and two separate squadron messes and an officers' mess. The airdrome is a mile east of the camp past an old aqua duct built by the Romans, still carrying water. The airdrome has one long east-west strip in the process of being lengthened; a tar-covered strip with crushed rock lay down by hand. A landing strip would be more than a mile long with a number of taxi paths leading off of it."[1]

Headquarters for the unit was located in an olive grove

a mile away from the living quarters. A large tent was set up in front of the mess hall with long wooden tables placed end to end to use as serving lines. The mess tent, as it was known, was located so far away from the central area of the camp that the walk back and forth two or three times a day took up a large part of the men's time, often making them wonder if it was better to go hungry. (This separation was maintained in the interest of sanitation.) When the group was on the move, C rations and K rations were eaten. C rations consisted of six small cans, three for meat and three for bread. The units were marked M for meat and B for bread and could be eaten hot or cold. M units, for example, consisted of meat and beans, meat and vegetables, and meat and potatoes.

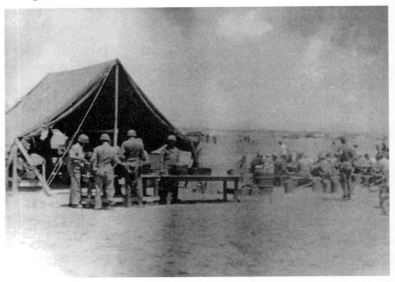

Mess tent at unit Headquarters

K rations were developed for paratroopers. They were packaged in lightweight containers and consisted of 8,300 calories; ninety-nine grams of this caloric count came from protein. These rations were labeled breakfast, lunch, and dinner. All meals also included the grit of the desert in the teeth and the spitting out of bugs.

Besides the stifling heat, windstorms, and sand, the men also had to endure flies and sand fleas. There was no relief from the awful fleas, and being bitten constantly made a difficult living situation even worse. Because of the insect issue, the men often kept their shirts and long pants on despite the horrible heat. They learned to endure the dirt, sleeping on a cot under mosquito netting, living with no showers and poor food. In spite of these conditions at Berguent Airfield, the aircrews were still expected to perform at maximum efficiency.

"The Bright spot at Berguent," reads an entry in the 50th War Diary, "was the swimming pool, which had been erected about two miles from the field the previous summer by a battalion of French engineers. The terrific African heat was in a small way relieved by the cooling waters of this pool, and the entire personnel spent a considerable part of their time washing not only themselves but their clothing in the waters from this delightfully cooling pool with its ever-changing water fed by Artesian wells."[2]

In June, the group moved to Field "J," five miles northwest of Kairouan, Tunisia. This was the second Field the Ninth Air Force called home. Here, "split trenches had to be dug and an effective guard system established, all of which were accomplished in a creditably short period. A ring of anti-aircraft artillery was installed by British forces and the entire area took on a somewhat forbiddingly warlike appearance.[3]

Lamb wrote home that his living situations were pretty rough, especially after an African rain. The mud was horrible. He also noted how busy his days were. He was healthy, brown as an Indian, taking a vitamin daily, and getting into better shape. There was little to spend money on. The morale of the men was good, except when they heard the Nazis broadcasting about the mine strikes. It made the men furious, but they realized everyday what a wonderful place the United States was to live, so the rumors and propaganda did not affect them much. Lamb requested that his family send letters airmail because they would arrive a month earlier than those coming through the Army channels.

On Sunday, June 20, 1943, Lamb wrote his mother:

> Today is Sunday, but it's just about like any other day here. Pat Fowlkes, our chaplain, an Episcopalian from Richmond, held services, but I was too busy to go. The church consists of the rear end of my ambulance, which opens up and can be used as an altar. Attendance is very good usually. Pat is one of the finest men I've ever known, a man whom I consider as the kind of person a preacher should be. His wife, Betty knows her, is to have a baby in August. She went to Hollins. Pat and I spend a great deal of time together, as we visit the hospitals and wounded usually together. He is 28. I am quite well these days, in spite of everything. Some parts of this country are not too bad, but I'm afraid we weren't so lucky, as this place is the worst I've ever seen, could be worse off than we are however. I've been busy, as the other doctor in my outfit has been seriously ill. He is some better now, thou. Needless to say how much I miss you all and how much I think of you. I live almost entirely for the future and the time when we can all be together again. The mine strikes cause quite a bit of discussion and hatred here.

Weather was as much a factor in Tunisia as it was in

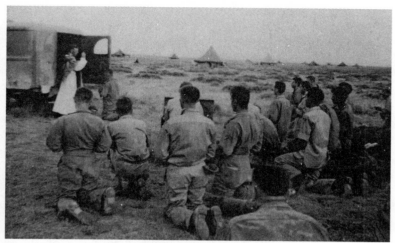

Church service performed out of an ambulance

Monaco. This account was given by a crewman on July 23, 1943:

> A major wind and rain storm hit the camp. It became necessary for everyone to hang onto their tents. Meanwhile, they watch everything not tied down fly away. The planes were heavy enough to remain on the ground but the gliders were not. The glider planes flew on their own. They looped, rolled and performed amazing movements and fell to the ground, then a pile of junk. Two gliders flew in perfect formation, soared high side by side, and crashed on the ground in the same position.[4]

Service in the Army Air Forces was unique. Pulitzer Prize-winning journalist Ernie Pyle offers this insight in his book *Brave Men*:

> I had to make some psychological adjustments when I switched from the infantry . . . A man approached death rather decently in the Air Forces. He died well-fed and clean-

shaven, if that was any comfort. He was at the front only a few hours of the day, instead of day and night for months on end. . . . He still had some acquaintance with an orderly life, even though he might be living in a tent. But in the infantry a soldier had to become half beast in order to survive.[5]

Air Force troop carrier crews consisted of five members: the pilot, co-pilot, navigator, crew chief, and radio operator. Sometimes a radar operator would also be aboard. Navigators were responsible for keeping the plane on course and were in short supply. Many times only the lead plane would have one as a member of the crew. The crew chief saw that the plane remained in top flying condition and gave instructions to the paratroopers. The radio operator maintained communications with the ground controller and saw to cargo and supplies.

The rate of survival for a combat crew was only twenty missions. This reality damaged morale and a crew's ability to do its job, for the fear of dying loomed large. By 1943, one tour of duty was mandated. After each pilot flew twenty-five missions, he was rotated back to the States and reassigned to train new pilots.

Lamb flew missions to observe work conditions of the crew. By using these observations, he could offer suggestions on how to improve the work environment. Since he was not a pilot himself, Lamb did not qualify for the rotation program back home, which meant he would not see his family for years.

Troop carrier crews and glider pilots flew unarmed planes and gliders low and deep into enemy territory through heavy flak. Their mission, with standing orders not to take evasive action, was to deliver personnel and supplies. Missions were often flown at sunrise and sunset so that pilots could use the sun as a blind, bringing planes out of the sun to prevent them from being seen. Evening missions created constant concern because of the high number of crash landings that occurred from lack of visibility. In one serious C-47 crash, the plane came off the runway and climbed nicely. It pulled up sharply, stalled, and the left wing dipped sharply, and then plummeted straight down. Smoked billowed, and no one survived.

All planned missions began with pilot briefings. During the meeting, an account of the events of the last twenty-four hours was given. The briefing would include what was happening in England, Russia, and Africa. Seeing the bigger picture and knowing they were not isolated helped to keep up the morale of the men.

Before the pilots left for a flight they were served high-carbohydrate meals such as cookies and coffee to keep their energy up and keep them alert. When the planes "rolled out" or left on a mission, the tension was heavy around the camp.

The Army Air Forces trained with the British in desert flying. The British had been fighting in North Africa before the United States entered the war, so the Royal Air Force's knowledge and expertise was of value to the US pilots. Airmen and paratroopers were trained in Tunisia in preparation for the invasion of Sicily. In Africa, missing the drop zone was an ongoing problem and would continue to be an issue throughout the war.

Thorough training was essential to preventing as many casualties and failed missions as possible. This account was given in the June 1943 to August 1943 record in the 50th War Diary: "An intensive training program had been set up and was religiously followed by all personnel of the squadron at Berguent. The ships made various trips to Casablanca to haul squadron tools to the new base, in addition to training with the 82nd Airborne Division which was the chief duty at this station. Sometime [sic] was spent in training with gliders."

Lamb, along with the rest of the ground crew, was left behind to wait anxiously for the planes' return from a mission, knowing full well that some of them would not make it back. Plane crews were not only fellow airmen but in many cases friends. Lamb stayed busy with his duties, hoping to divert his mind from worries over whether or not his pilots and their crews would arrive home safely.

With the squadron out on a mission, Lamb took care of odd jobs in camp. Base sanitation was his responsibility, which often included inspecting the latrines. If other men were busy, the job of cleaning them fell to Lamb as well. He also had to review the mess tent sanitation practices as meals were prepared and plates and utensils were cleaned. The potential for food contamination by bugs was high, so fly traps were set up and food storage containers were often inspected. Lamb had to make sure the local cooks were not sick and were safely handling the food and using correct cooking temperatures and methods. "There was plenty of food," Lamb said, "but it wasn't always good."

Proper garbage disposal practices were important to maintaining the camp's health, and Lamb maintained the garbage pit to deter insects and prevent disease. The water supply likewise required monitoring. It was necessary to

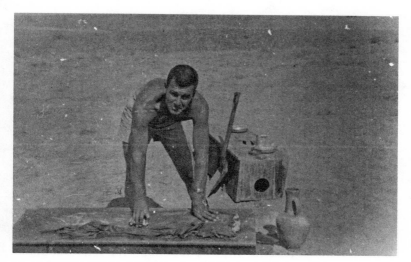

Lamb cleaning a camp latrine

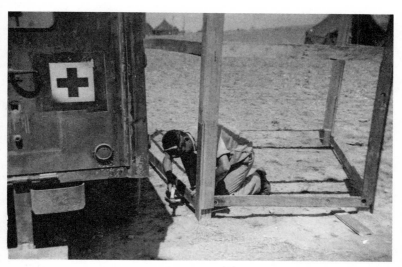

Lamb building a shower

keep the Lyster bags that held the drinking water clean. The lack of water in the area created poor sanitary conditions that contributed to medical issues.

There were medical and squadron reports to fill out monthly. Lamb not only reported to the flight commander but also to the flight surgeon in the higher echelon. This fight surgeon served as adviser on human factors and policy matters such as tours of duty, rest, and rotations. Lamb was responsible for recording emergency statistics. Medical reports would go up channels to be sent to the Library of Congress, making them available for congressional review. On December 31, Lamb filled out an annual report that went to the surgeon general showing the quantity of all medical-department supplies.

Medical supplies and equipment had been scarce in 1942 and 1943. The rapid buildup of the Army left it unprepared to handle the supply demand, and inexperienced personnel often did not properly handle, pack, or label the materials. Until early 1944, the theater surgeon department seldom filled medical supply requisitions. Instead, this was done through the Service of Supply (SOS). However, because the SOS was so inefficient, the theater surgeon's office circumvented them and delivered supplies through Newark, New Jersey. By 1944, the SOS was reorganized and became known as Army Service Forces. Medical supplies were then the responsibility of the theater surgeon exclusively.

While medical staff had experienced difficulties in the early years of the war, Lamb luckily experienced no shortages of medical supplies. By the time he arrived overseas, the need to keep the Air Forces well-supplied was understood. Commanders of medical supply depots tended to disregard regulations and sent items "peculiar to the AAF" with efficiency. This did not please other branches of the Army.

Standard medical supplies included drugs, dressings, instruments, diagnostic and laboratory equipment, furniture, linen and bedding for the clinic, mess equipment and supplies, cleaning and preserving supplies, stationery and office supplies, and field equipment. Requisition forms were required to replace supplies used. General inventory reports were filed in March and September while reports for non-deteriorating items were filed quarterly.

The camp would break into a flurry of activity when the alert came that the planes were returning from a mission. Of the planes that did return, many came in shot up and limping onto the runway. This created a serious danger. If a plane's landing gear failed, it would inevitably crash nose down or skid on its belly, which often cost lives. Even if the planes had not experienced any damage in the air, landing could still prove tricky. Engine failures also led to crashes and crew deaths. Lamb assisted the doctors of other Groups during emergency landings. There were two to three doctors per wing of the Ninth Air Force.

Many times, twelve planes would leave and only half or fewer would return. After this type of mission, the entire camp was affected emotionally. Sometimes the returning pilots could report what had happened and where the lost planes went down, but at other times they had no idea what occurred. The missing planes were designated as "missing in action." It was part of Lamb's responsibility to file the missing air crew reports.

Due to the number of men that were lost, replacements

were constantly joining the wing. Lamb met with the new combat crew members to discuss their current medical issues, potential problems and prevention, and things to be concerned about while living in the desert.

Lamb advanced toward the front a day or two after paratroopers were dropped during an invasion. He moved with the Army, working when the pilots worked and resting when they rested, sometimes going three to four days without sleep.

A typical bad day for Lamb would include constant activity, often beginning before dawn. As this log-book record demonstrates, a flight surgeon's work ranged from sick bay visits, filling out paperwork, and even just being available for his men if they needed to talk.

0400 Up early for briefing at Group-coffee and crackers there. Paratrooper and supply drop, short 2 planes. Weather poor. After briefing, check oxygen equipment myself for the 2 new crews.

0500 In the ambulance on the line for takeoff. There are only 2 of us on duty-another is off at school somewhere and the group surgeon is at a meeting. Write a quick letter home.

0515 Called to sick bay. Lt. Marsh carried in by his crewmen, too weak to climb into the aircraft-Diarrhea all night-Bad cow?-Too much whiskey?-Or nerves? He's stayed in his hut smoking and drinking since the last flight when his buddy got a direct hit and crashed. Crew looked relieved when I grounded him, and the sergeant made out the hospital ticket.

0540 One of ours-Capt. Martin lost power on takeoff-crashed into the Mediterranean and burned-Poor devils!

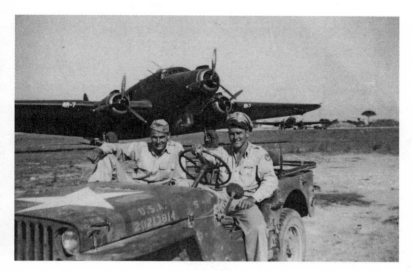

Lamb (driver's side) with another member of the 50th TCS in front of a C-47

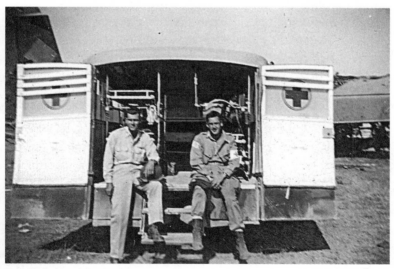

Lamb (left) with an aide

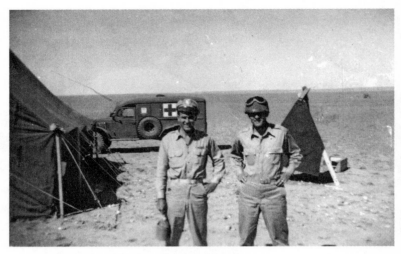

Lamb (left) with a member of the 50th TCS

Air-sea went there quick but no survivors. One of the new crews lost an engine half-way down the field-skidded off the runway and nosed over gently. No one hurt but the navigator who broke an arm when he jumped out-sergeant-puts a temporary splint on him; and I take the pilot who's shaking bad to my quarters for a few stiff drinks-When he relaxes, I give him a second and my driver takes him to his hut. Lucky!

0630 Everyone airborne–to breakfast.

0700 Sick call: 2 or 3 men with bronchitis (or malaria, or diarrhea) to overcrowd the already full dispensary. Couple of fellows getting edgy-headaches-dizzy spell: gave them appointments to come back later for a little quiet talk. Usual dressings-all o.k. Sergeant and I work on the reports. Reports!

0930 The other flight surgeon and I flip to see who will stick around for the cripples and the aborts so my driver and I start off for visit to the hospital. It is already over 100 degrees . . .

1000 Station Hospital men in surgery doing fine, except Lt. Rollins who has minor flak wound in abdomen-says he can't eat. Talked with him half an hour or so-his crew has ditched twice and somebody had been hurt on every one of their 10 missions-I think he's had it and suggested to the ward officer that he'd do better in the general hospital-he won't be fit to fly for months.

1100 The major called me to his office and raised hell about one of our men who went AWOL during the night- the kid is a ground crewmen that I sent in with acute amebic dysentery-we're not permitted to treat him in the dispensary now! I'd seen the kid on the flight line the morning before and wondered how he got out so soon. Some guys . . .

1200 Lunch at the hospital. Picked up some stuff from the pharmacy and from medical supply-very generous fellows . . .

1300 General hospital. Several of our mob got in here when they got lost in a surprise sandstorm, and crashed nearby. Doctor on the officer's wanted to talk to me about the pilot, Capt. Stephens who it seems is very morose, won't talk about the war, his family, or anything for that matter. His broken ribs and chest injuries are doing all right, but the doc has requested a psychiatric consultation. I told him to forget it-B's always quiet, and of course he feels bad about smashing up his plane-she's always been lucky until that trip. He only thinks about planes and women and won't talk much about either of them-He's an iron man and his crew idolizes him-he needs a psychiatrist like I do-the young doctor is not convinced and we have quite a debate-says he knows when a man is cracking up. I say wait a bit, let me talk to Stephens. I'll manage to get Stephens out before they do anything drastic . . .

1400 Sat in on a Disposition Board involving some of our men-what a riot! One of our mechanics with headaches that they said was hostile to his lieutenant-they think he better be sent back. I know better: his headaches are hangovers from the rotten moonshine he and his pals are making somewhere on the base-we'll probably lose him even though he's a good mechanic, overhung or not.

1430 On the way back to the field passed our ambulance-stopped-four of our men with fairly serious injuries from flak and a crash when their cripple came in-not too bad, but too much for our sick bay to handle . . .

1500 Talked with men with nerves-one had a "Dear John" letter which I had to read-the other just needed someone to talk to-He'll be all right with some phenobarb and a little more rest-twelve hours a day, seven days a week in the shops can get a little rugged for some of the boys-The last man, navigator is worried about his ability to do his job-he's loused up a couple of trips and they got back because of plain dumb luck-I can't make out whether he's stupid, or beginning to crack up-we'll talk some more tomorrow . . .

1610 Back in the ambulance on the line, "sweating out" the returns as the fog begins to roll in . . . Our radio brings us all the chatter between the tower and the planes. Priority in landing goes to the planes with wounded men aboard-there are only 2 this time, they get down safely-moderate flak and machine gun wounds which can be patched up when we get all the planes in-The other gets its wheels down so we all raced over to the crash strip, and ran along with her as she came in-a messy landing-cartwheel, then caught on fire. The crash crew got there first and had foam on her and we got all the men but the copilot who was pinned in debris. We were working on him when the gun belts started to go, and then the fire started again in the cabin so we couldn't get back-the radioman said he died on the way in, and that's the way it looked to me, the few seconds I had to see him. Two other planes missing-one was seen going down over the target-no one knew what happened to the other. According to my information it was a little worse than average for a tough mission-but not bad considering . . .

1700 Help serve at the aircrew bar after interrogation-all who feel the need of medicinal whiskey get it courtesy of the Air Surgeon bless him! No one very edgy, except LT. Thompson who has just lost the second roommate in two weeks-Later at the bar I played gin rummy with him and we philosophized about luck and life and things . . .

1730 Dinner-the mess is getting worse-food too greasy-mess attendant not too clean-the kitchen will get a thorough inspection-the mess sergeant will get chewed tomorrow . . .

1830 Made rounds in the dispensary with my partner-everyone doing well, thanks to sulfa, paregoric and phenobarb-Only a few there for evening sick call-a special one that I run for the men who are too busy on the line for the regular one-Sergeant and I write up the reports on the day's casualties-Crash crew brought in the body from the burned plane-described the wounds-he may have been dead when they crashed-made out the report, tagged the body and it off to the hospital for pronounce of death, then to the graves people . . .

1930 Back to the General Hospital for a medical meeting-the wing Surgeon thinks we should all be there-and attendance required, one goes-Not a bad clinic on hepatitis and frostbit-some good ideas-there was a social hour afterwards and I ran into a classmate that just came over . . .

2300 Back home-and to bed-too tired to write home.

0200 Sergeant wakened me-one of the men has DT's and is sitting in his hut shooting the snakes with his 45. I took the gun away for him, and we got him to the sick bay where some IV Amytal finally put him out and so to bed again.[6]

Chapter Three
Medicine

To properly care for aviation personnel, flight surgeons specialized in diagnosing and treating medical issues particular to pilots and ground crews. Lamb regularly tended to men who complained of vertigo and nausea while flying, conditions that would ground a pilot. He became familiar with specific vision problems, such as a difficulty adjusting to flying in the dark after exposure to the bright light of an explosion. Sometimes illness would strike when there was a lull in the fighting or when pilots were grounded by bad weather. Since they were so accustomed to the adrenaline rush of flying, pilots could easily be stressed by excess down time. The crews would spent this time in the camp talking about girls, rumors, their experiences back home and in the air, their hopes for life after the war, and their opinions of the officers. Sometimes a casual remark might be made about what happens when a man dies.

When planes landed at the field after a mission, the injured men became Lamb's primary focus. He, along with his aides, conducted triage, prioritizing the men from the most seriously wounded to those who could wait for care. Using this process, Lamb determined which evacuees needed to be sent to the hospital while efficiently treating less-serious injuries himself, which allowed for the best allocation of his resources.

Wounds to the abdomen, head, or chest were beyond Lamb's capabilities and limited equipment. Most of the men with these types of injuries were immediately taken to the hospital as transportation allowed. The amount of time that elapsed from injury to arrival at the hospital often made the difference between life and death. Emergency medical tags were attached to the men, usually over the chest or as near as possible, to indicate their name, unit of service, full diagnosis, and the treatment given.

Often organs and tissue had shifted out of place or no longer existed. Many times there was nothing visible for Lamb to recognize from his medical school anatomy class. Flight surgeon medicine was not the clean, sterile medicine that Lamb had practiced in the controlled environment of a hospital. Instead it was blood spurting through torn clothes, broken bones, and deep tissue ripped away by white-hot fragments that caused the body to be red, twisted, and mangled. Arms, legs, muscles, tendons, stomachs, and intestines were slashed open by flak and shrapnel. A head injury from a crash landing often meant death. While Lamb and his aides worked and quietly spoke to an injured man on the runway, men around them were running and shouting as they worked to save lives by putting out a burning plane or moving a damaged one off the runway so another could land.

Men moaned in agony as Lamb and his aides hurried to stop bleeding, concentrating on the arms, legs, neck, and face. Immobilizing torn tissues, treating shock, controlling hemorrhaging, and preventing loss of limb meant quick and adequate control of bleeding. Clothes were cut away and tourniquets applied and then released in order to determine where the bleeding vessel was located, which was often difficult to identify because of the destruction of the skin and muscle in the area. A pressure bandage was applied to stem the flow of blood before suturing.

The double-pole, eight-foot-long canvas litters that were used to carry men were often stained from blood. A Neil Robertson litter, designed to move a person from a tight space while supporting his back, was used to remove the injured from planes. Constructed of semi-rigid canvas, it was wrapped around the patient mummy-fashion, giving him enough support to be lowered vertically.

If there was an ambulance available, something Lamb did not always have access to, the injured were carried to the dispensary in a litter. Army ambulances carried four stretchers each or nine sitting wounded. The ambulances were equipped with two-way radios and were often referred to as "meat wagons."

The less-severely injured were laid out on the ground until the worst injuries had been cared for. Under Lamb's direction, these injured crewmen were sent to the dispensary, which would be a large canvas tent or an area located below ground level that blended in with the surrounding terrain, camouflaged in order to protect it from enemy air raids. There, airmen were further triaged and injuries identified. Lamb's aides handled routine bandaging of less serious wounds and the splinting of sprains and broken bones. The wounded who did not leave on the first trucks or airplanes were stabilized, bandaged, and kept comfortable until later evacuation to the hospital in the rear. (For a more detailed discussion of the chain of evacuation and the types of hospitals established during the war, see chapter nine.)

Lamb performed no major surgery on site. The most seriously injured would be sent to a hospital behind the front lines. The injuries of even the worst accident victims brought into a city emergency room could not compare to the combat wounds Lamb saw. Simple stitching and surgery had been a part of his internship training, but repairing gaping chest wounds and amputating limbs had not. Deceased soldiers were also sent to a hospital where they were officially pronounced dead and paperwork was completed. The bodies were then returned to their group for burial. Lamb did not do any legal pronouncing of death.

When Lamb joined the war in Africa, hospitals were normally located three to fifteen miles behind the front lines. Prior to late 1943, however, the hospitals could have been hundreds of miles away, even in a different country from where the fighting was taking place. These rear-line field surgical hospitals were the predecessor to the Mobile Army Surgical Hospital (M.A.S.H.) units.

While recuperating, the men made the most of being in the hospital. They returned to their groups eager to talk about how much they enjoyed having soap to bathe with and hot tomato soup to eat—a real treat.

At the front, the only medical intervention available to support life was plasma, adrenaline, caffeine, and morphine. Plasma infusions were given to ward off shock and were administered through a large needle placed in a viable vein, if one could be located. Too much plasma could produce edema or tissue swelling, causing the wounded's lungs to froth. Unlike whole blood, plasma was stored in cans and required no refrigeration, making it much more accessible. All blood transfusions were done at the hospital, and blood was in short supply.

For Lamb, burns were common injuries. Vaseline-covered gauze that contained an antiseptic was used to cover the damaged skin. The gauze came in prepackaged packs and was a standard supply in a flight surgeon's clinic. Sulfanilamide powder was used on the initial dressing and subsequent redressing of wounds. Carried as powder or tablets in first aid kits during a mission, it was actively used in Lamb's dispensary. Ironically, the value of sulfur powder for treating wounds was taken from the Germans.

Morphine was normally given as a local anesthetic and used to keep the patient quiet. Later in the war it could be administered by pre-measured injectable syrettes. An injured man could even use it on himself before reaching medical help. The solider had to be careful not to overdose; therefore the amount of morphine was controlled. A large "M" was placed on the foreheads of the men who had received morphine so they would not be given additional doses at the hospital. Also available were codeine, paregoric, bismuth, and sulfaguanidine. Novocaine was most commonly used to ease pain from sprained ankles.

Penicillin was not widely used until late 1943, having been only recently discovered. Lamb had no access to other antibiotics while in North Africa, and penicillin was the answer to numerous infection problems for both the wounded and those with venereal disease. The antibiotic came in glass vials and was administered by syringe. Sulfa drugs, penicillin, blood plasma, and the portability of whole blood were all innovations in medicine during World War II. The supplies found in the canvas medical pouch that Lamb regularly carried with him included black, hard-rubber vials, a litter-carrying strap, adhesive plaster, a field tourniquet, hypodermic set with sterilizer, bandage scissors, bandages (both compression and triangular), absorbent cotton, a lead pencil and eraser, safety pins, three types of forceps, gauze, silk-braided sutures, surgical needles, thermometer, morphine syrettes, iodine swabs, ammonia, a book of emergency medical tags, sulfanilamide in powder and pill form, a burn injury set, eye dressing set, two operating knives, and sharp pointed scissors.

These same items could be in found in Lamb's clinic. Instruments were stored in jars of bichloride of mercury for sterilization. Plastic gloves were not readily available outside of hospitals, so flight surgeons and their aides would normally be forced to use their bare hands. Hospitals used chloroform to put their patients to sleep, but Lamb used hydrochloride. Suturing, however, was performed without any type of anesthesia. Medical staff used portable surgical lamps on small tripod stands for light; on the airfield at night, headlights and flashlights were an additional help.

Lamb's cases were all recorded in a log book: patient name, serial number, rank, date, time, and diagnosis. Along with two to five aides, there were also a dentist and a member of the clergy assigned to Lamb's group.

Another important aspect of the flight surgeon's duty was to handle public health and preventative medicine. When Lamb was not caring for the wounded or handling

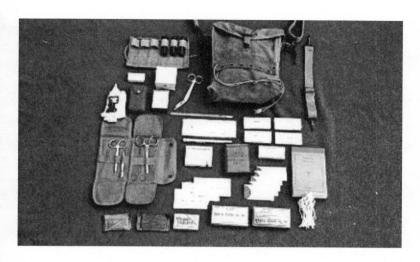

Flight surgeon's medical pack and supplies

minor cuts and routine infections, his attention turned to
seeing that the men remained healthy enough to fly. Twice
a year he would give lectures on the importance of good
hygiene. Lamb's only familiarity with many of the diseases
he faced came from textbooks. In some instances, he had not
actually seen a case of the disease before joining the military.
He often had to study the symptoms of these diseases in
order to diagnose and treat the men. Flight surgeons were
issued technical manuals such as *Military Chemistry and
Chemical Agents, Scrub Typhus Fever, Avoidance of Relapse of
Vivax Malaria by Use of Suppressive Medication,* and *Guides
to Therapy for Medical Officers.* At different times during the
war, Lamb was also provided field manuals: *The Army
Leg Splint; Transportation of the Sick and Wounded, Splints,
Appliances and Bandages; Defense Against Chemical Attack;*
and *Operations in Cold and Extreme Snow,* for example.

Lamb's primary written guideline was the Flight Surgeon Handbook. Light blue in color, the paperback book was eight by ten inches and three-fourths of an inch thick. It contained information compiled at the School of Aviation Medicine: tables and measurements to use daily in selection of flying personnel, diagnostic procedures, Army regulations regarding examinations, short summaries of diseases, procedures for using supplies, tips for effective administration and sanitation, and guidelines for practicing medicine during combat.

Venereal disease was one of the largest health issues of the war. Syphilis and gonorrhea counts among men rose at an alarming rate after the men went overseas. Education was stressed, abstinence encouraged, and condoms handed out. Condoms were the most realistic prevention method. Lamb gave compulsory group lectures that, in reality, had very little effect. The majority of the local women (prostitutes or not) was infected with one venereal disease or another. It was estimated that 50 percent of the local women had VD and 95-100 percent of the prostitutes in large cities were infected.

Lamb had to perform regular "short arm inspections" on the men. The enlisted men were roused from bed at 4:30 a.m. to 5:00 a.m. by the barracks sergeant yelling, "Drop your cock and grab your socks!" Men would line up in front of their bunks while Lamb and one of his aides would go down the ranks ordering the men to "milk it." The men would then squeeze their penises from the base to the tip. If a white milky substance was present then the man had gonorrhea.

The availability of penicillin had a major impact in

improving the VD situation. In 1942, there was zero production of penicillin ampoules. Mass production started in 1943 with only 7,500 ampoules manufactured in the year, but by 1944 this number had increased to 10,276,000. Administrating shots as treatment was outlined in the Flight Surgeon Handbook.

Desert living brought on unique medical issues. Sunburn was one of the obvious problems that had to be attended. Insects caused illness in varying degrees that often became major problems. Fleas created the largest health crisis in Africa, though sand flea bites also made sleeping very uncomfortable.

Typhus, a bacterial disease spread by lice, became an epidemic in North Africa due to poor sanitation and the decay of refuse and the dead. The men with typhus would come down with chills, cough, and fever. Delousings of civilian and military personnel and the areas around the camps by dusting with DDT were performed regularly.

In the wet and rainy northern coast of Africa, mosquitoes transmitted malaria, grounding the pilots and keeping other crew members away from their jobs with chills and fever. Malaria was treated by quinacrine hydrochloride or quinine. It was rationed four times a week and intense instruction on sanitation was given, which involved food preparation, water purification, and waste disposal. Yellow fever was another disease caused by mosquitoes that Lamb had to treat. A viral infection common to the desert region of Africa, this infection has no known cure and causes heart problems, bleeding, and could put a patient into a coma. Lamb gave yellow fever shots to the group as a whole. He held a clinic and saw that each man was inoculated. Mosquitoes were also responsible for a disease that caused the scrotum to swell to a horribly large size. It was commonly called a "wheelbarrow full of scrotum" by the men. This disease made them particularly miserable.

Other diseases that Lamb treated in Africa were pneumonia, tuberculosis, diphtheria, relapsing fever, dengue fever, hepatitis, scabies, cholera, beriberi, smallpox, leprosy, ringworm, hookworms, yaws, bilharzia, heat stroke, and foot problems. Sanitation, food storage, and lack of clean water and refrigeration caused food poisoning and amoebic dysentery. Sulfaguanadine, paregoric, and bismuth were used to treat these problems.

Locals were hired to dig latrines and trenches, cook and clean, or help with whatever was needed in camp. Lamb also saw to their care. He used green disinfectant soap, medicines, and common sense to treat diseases. Health campaign posters were produced by the surgeon general, and Lamb posted these to remind men of preventive measures they should take to avoid contracting diseases.

Beyond general healthcare, Lamb's paramount responsibility was to keep the planes in the air by seeing to the pilots' well-being and by assessing their ability to carry out the special duties required during each mission. It was Lamb's burden to form a diagnosis, plan treatment, and decide if the pilots were fit for duty and well enough to return to flying. Evaluating whether or not a pilot was fit for flying consisted of determining the type of duty the flyer would be assigned — based on the number of missions he could tolerate and the extent to which his efficiency was

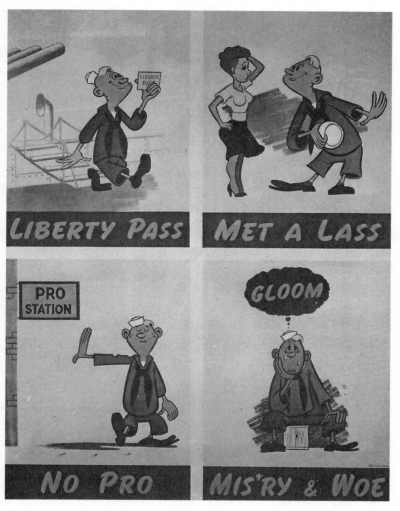

VD poster issued by the surgeon general (Courtesy National Archives Still Picture Branch)

impaired — and how dangerous he would be to his crew. The fight surgeon's obligation was to enable the command to get the maximum effort out of all flight personnel.

After a mission, stress and nervous problems often affected a pilot's ability to sleep, leaving him on edge or alert all night. If this was the case, Lamb or the pilot's commanding officer could make the decision to ground the man. A pilot's emotional problems could affect personal safety and his ability to handle the weight of responsibility required to protect the lives of his crew. Frequently there was conflict between an individual's medical condition and needs and the commander's demand to have a full flight crew. This put Lamb in an undesirable position. In this situation, his diplomacy skills and his relationship with both the pilot and the commander became invaluable.

Mental tension was a problem when crews were overworked. Pilots were considered temperamental, intelligent, glamour boys addicted to adrenaline rushes. They were highly trained, almost irreplaceable, and required a more tender hand when they had issues. These characteristics often complicated the symptoms of fatigue. Lamb made the judgment call as to whether or not a crew member was suffering from "flying fatigue." After long or intense periods of flying time and repeated missions with little rest, aircrews' efficiency noticeably declined. This normally occurred when pilots had passed a hundred hours of flying, or fifteen to twenty hours at one time. Fatigue manifested itself in nervous disorders from the abnormal strain on an individual. Symptoms included hyper-vigilance (or being ever on alert), staleness, headache, insomnia, gastrointestinal disturbances, anxiety, phobic reactions, irritability, regressive reactions, and difficulties in forming and keeping relationships. A fatigued man wore a "haggard and weary expression or none at all," would laugh or joke around only little if at all, was listless, and had a small appetite. During a physical examination, issues such as increased pulse rate, tremors, and abnormal breathing would become apparent. Exhaustion was often the cause of insubordination, excessive drinking, and the inability to concentrate. The nature of the strain depended on the personality of the individual and the intensity of the fatigue.

Pilot error due to flying fatigue accounted for most flight-related casualties. Throughout the war, new procedures were regularly devised to diagnose the problem. Fatigue from coming down after an adrenaline rush such as that caused by flying also had to be addressed. Sleep and rest were extremely important in battling flying fatigue, as was maintaining a proper diet and healthy weight.

Ernie Pyle wrote about this issue in *Brave Men*:

> A soldier who has been a long time in the line does have a "look" in his eyes that anyone who knows about it can discern. It's a look of dullness, eyes that look without seeing, eyes that see without conveying that is the display room for what lies behind it—exhaustion, lack of sleep, tension for too long, weariness that is too great, fear beyond fear, misery to the point of numbness, a look of suppressing indifference to anything anybody can do. It's a look I dread to see on men.

> And yet to me it's one of the perpetual astonishments of a war life that human beings recover as quickly as they do. For example, a unit may be pretty well exhausted, but if they are lucky enough to be blessed with some sunshine and warmth they'll begin to be normal after two days out of the line. The human spirit is just like a cork.[1]

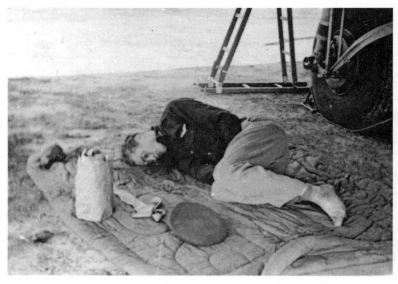

Pilot sleeping under a plane after a long day, North Africa

In the early years of the war, there were no policies established for handling psychiatric casualties. Flight surgeons were required to distinguish between true cowardice and the lack of courage, which would cause a man to refuse to fly. Lack of courage could be caused by stress, concern for family, or loss of a close comrade. Skillfully, Lamb had to determine the source of the problem and the effective treatment based on how well he knew the individual. After an emergency landing, a pilot often froze up when landing the next time. The anxiety would develop from a creditable amount of emotional trauma or stress. No disciplinary action was taken when this was thought to be the case, though the "ground shyness" did have to be worked through. It was important for a pilot to learn to relax and regain his confidence in his abilities.

Lamb had two main methods of preventing or delaying

combat-related stress symptoms. One was to regularly test the men's psychological health; the other was to develop a personal relationship with the men. A crewman needed someone who understood his problems, was responsive to his needs, and was under the same command. Lamb was encouraged by his superiors to put himself among the pilots and work with them regularly; this is was an important step toward earning their trust so they would take his advice when he told them they were sick or needed to be hospitalized.

As the "doc," Lamb had to be everything to the men — their general practitioner and at times their mother and father, spiritual guide, social director, and psychiatrist all wrapped up in one person. Lamb's particular soft-spoken bedside manner became invaluable in this area of the flight surgeon's duty. He was well-liked by the men. It was believed that it took at least three years of close contact with the pilots to develop the skills to handle their problems most effectively. It is not surprising that being a flight surgeon was a difficult job.

As the war lengthened, the importance of friendships and rapid return to duty after rest treatment was recognized. Members of an aircrew or squadron personnel developed a team mentality that required mutual interdependence, responsibility, and loyalty. Each squadron lived in a separate area and formed distinct families. For a mission, they fused into one big group. Planes and men lost to the enemy and the sea caused morale problems. It was difficult for the men to do their jobs after such a loss, and it was rare not to have causalities. Capt. Emmett Allamon, a regimental surgeon, referred to this as "mental wreckage."

Belief in continued life — a peaceful and orderly world

where death and destruction were not the daily goals — was necessary to keep a man's morale high. The mental health of the pilots and ground crews depended on reasonable leave policies, which involved time at special Army Air Forces rest centers or camps. Men who completed twenty missions or more often lost their positive outlook and needed to be refreshed. The idea that "nothing can happen to me" was replaced by "something horrible will happen to me." Lamb could prescribe phenobarbital and Benzedrine, but there was little else he could do in these cases except talk to the man, see that he got some rest leave, and hope for the best.

Some men were admitted to a hospital's narcosis unit for a short stay. Few went to a general hospital, but most stayed in the dispensary or went to flight-surgeon-supervised rest camps. These rest camps were all planned in advance. The US Air Force had learned of their necessity from the Royal Air Force. The judicious use of rest leave was a powerful way of maintaining morale and combat effectiveness during World War II. At a rest camp, a man could take off his uniform, sleep late, and spend idle, lazy days. It was a place to retreat for a week or two and combat the hopelessness of feeling expendable. The men would gain weight, relax, and regain their self-confidence. Rest camps were one of the most important and successful parts of the "care for the flyer" program. In Africa, they were located in the coastal town of Oran, Algeria, and in Ain Taya, an area outside of Algiers, Algeria.

The men feared not being able to return to their group if they were gone from their job too long. It was important to them and the efficiency of the group to return as soon as possible. Lamb could keep a man on sick report in the dispensary for ninety-six hours to a week as a rule. If an airman remained in a hospital for more than thirty days, he was sent to an Air Force replacement depot. There was no assurance he would return to his group from the depot. The continuous influx of replacement crews was emotionally difficult on the old men as well as the new. No one wanted to get to know the new men because they might not live through the next day. At one point there were only four of the original pilots left in Lamb's squadron.

Operational fatigue, later known as post-traumatic stress disorder, was the inability to carry out a job as ordered because of anxiety. A pilot would be permanently relieved of duty if the squadron leader and Lamb agreed he had operational fatigue. If he refused to fly without this diagnosis, he forfeited ninety days of pay.

A Section 8 referred to the number on the regulations concerning discharges for psychological illness. Lamb would watch pilots closely to make sure they were not dangerous to themselves or others. He would become concerned if he saw any signs of a possible breakdown, such as the inability of a co-pilot to lift his leg to the ladder of the plane. Lamb would then determine whether or not to remove the man from duty.

The "nothing wrong with him" man was given a physical and had lab tests done. The crewman remained grounded with the possibility of facing a court martial and, if convicted, the disgrace of being dishonorably discharged and living with the shame. Before leaving the States, the men were read the regulations about dishonorable discharges and consequences for going AWOL. With eight to ten months of expensive training invested in each flyer, the decision to dishonorably discharge a man was not to be made lightly. This judgment placed a tremendous responsibility on Lamb; in later years, an evaluation board would help handle this issue.

Lamb was entitled to his own R&R. He was given one night a week off and could go into town, if there was one nearby. Other doctors would be assigned to the group whenever he had to be gone any length of time. Because of the language barrier, he did not interact much with the locals. Lamb had been issued a revolver before leaving the States. He carried no weapon regularly, because it was forbidden by the Geneva Convention, but he did carry a pistol when he was out alone. Leave was given for men to go to Egypt and Palestine while the group was stationed in Africa. The pilots of the Ninth Air Force used a stripped-down plane the men called "the Mongrel" to travel to their R&R location.

Chapter Four
Sicily

The US Seventh Army, commanded by Gens. George Patton and Omar Bradley, led the invasion into Sicily from North Africa under the code name Operation Husky. The plan was for the Allies to take Sicily and work their way up the boot of Italy. This would remove Italy from the war and pull German troops away from the Russian front. As part of the invasion force, the Ninth Air Force took off from fields L and J in the Kairouan area of Tunisia on July 10, 1943. The 314th Troop Carrier Group (TCG), led by Quinn Corley and "Big" Joe McClure, were assigned to drop paratroopers from the 82nd Airborne Division into the vicinity of Gela on the southern coast of Sicily.

Because there were no distinguishing markings on US aircraft during the invasion of Sicily (like the black-and-white invasion stripes that would later be used during the Normandy landings), Allied soldiers on the ground and the US Navy shot down twenty-three American planes, mistaking them as enemy aircraft. Troop carrier planes were unarmed transports, putting them in an extremely dangerous position. The Ninth Air Force lost men and planes daily.

Bert Fernall, a member of the 45th Infantry Division, Anti-Aircraft Unit on the beach during the invasion, said

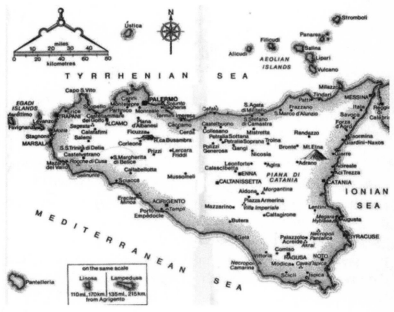

Sicily

that he and four other men had dug into the sand with their anti-aircraft gun. As planes flew overhead, they began shooting along with the other batteries set up on the beach. It was not until the airplanes had crashed into the water that they realized they were shooting down their own men. He and others attempted to save those men close enough to the beach, but many drowned trying to escape the plane or trapped under machinery. Sixty years later, Fernall cried over what had happened so many years ago as he stood on the beach in the spot where his foxhole had been located.

Never again did the United States attempt a complicated night navigation combat mission at low level through corridors of "friendly ships and friendly troops" with an armada of slow, vulnerable troop carrier aircraft.

A plane from the 314th TCG limped back to Africa, where it was discovered to have more than one hundred and forty holes put there by US Navy guns. The men at the field were amazed that it had managed to return. Marty Wolfe, a paratrooper during the invasion, later remembered, "The sound of bullets hitting a C-47 is something I'll never forget. It sounded a little like peas being dropped into a pot."

Each C-47 could tow a glider and hold twelve fully equipped paratroopers and two pilots. A carrier group could put 160 C-47s (or four squadrons) plus 160 gliders — or 320 gliders, if they were double towed — into the air at one time. The Horsa glider was a large plane with an eighty-eight-foot wingspan. At sixty-seven feet long, it weighed 8,400 pounds when empty. One glider could carry a 7,300 pound load. In addition to paratroopers, a typical load into combat would include a jeep, supplies, or even a bulldozer.

On the runway, the glider would be attached to the C-47. The glider pilot signaled to the mechanic that stood on the ground that he was ready and the ground crewmen passed the signal on to the radio man in the dome of the C-47. The tow plane rolled forward slowly as the slack was pulled out of the three-hundred-foot nylon tow rope. The C-47 pilot would then shove the throttles to their stops and the plane would lift into the air. At sixty-five miles per hour, the lighter-weight glider lifted off slowly. The glider pilot would then pull slightly above the C-47. After reaching eighty-five miles per hour, the C-47 and the glider would gain speed and altitude rapidly. When these tandems formed in the air for a mission, they would be overwhelming. One pilot commented that when he was in the middle of four planes and four glider elements—which together constituted one total element—he couldn't see the beginning or the end of the line from his position.

After reaching eighty-five miles per hour, the C-47 pilot would reach and maintain an altitude of one thousand feet and cruising speed of 160 miles per hour. This was done very carefully without flaps and without raising the nose to keep the airplanes slow and level. At this point, the glider pilot took his plane down below the C-47.

Slower speeds made controlling a C-47—holding the plane straight and level while being buffeted by prop wash from the neighboring planes—a difficult task. At this altitude it was cool and the plane shook. The glider received the same bucking and rocking from the propeller blast, but it improved when it moved below the C-47.

Near the drop zone, the C-47 would descend to five hundred feet. From there increasing power or throttling up was essential to hold and maintain a 120-miles-per-hour drop speed. A red light from the astrodome of the C-47 in front meant the drop zone was four minutes out; paratroopers stood and hooked up. As the paratroopers' jump zone was approached, a flashing green light signaled the time to jump. The paratroopers in the C-47 would stand and hook up to the temporary static line rigged up along the length of the plane. "Stand ready" was called. The paratroopers were all business as they went out the side door of the plane.

At the same time as these paratroopers were jumping, the

glider pilots landed in their designated locations and their load of paratroopers were piling out of the plane. Normally eighteen paratroopers were dropped from the C-47, but one of the problems that plagued the Army was how widely the paratroopers were scattered as they landed. The use of a glider allowed an additional eighteen men to land in the general vicinity of the dropped paratroopers, putting more than thirty men in the same area.

The C-47 pilot would make a slow, shallow turn over the landing area and then the glider pilot would pull a lever releasing the rope on the green light. The glider would leap away, allowing the C-47 to seemingly spring forward now that it was fifteen thousand pounds lighter.

At this point, the glider would be going ninety miles per hour and at an altitude of 1,200 feet. The pilot would check for smoke that would indicate wind direction. Taking the glider down to seventy miles per hour, the pilot would set up for the landing. He would then make three turns and at twenty feet begin to wait for impact.

The glider would touch down, and men would unload themselves and equipment as quickly as possible. It was crucial that the landing went well for a glider. Pilots moved their planes as far to the end of the target area as possible to avoid being hit by other landing gliders and maintain a two-hundred-foot distance between their plane and the next. All of this had to be accomplished while under enemy gun fire. The pilots dug in with the troopers and waited to be picked up, returned to base, and repeat the process all over again. The gliders were considered scrap and left behind.

The second combat mission for the IX Troop Carrier

Command occurred on July 11 at 1600 hours. Thirty planes, or three squadrons of the 314th, took off from L and J Fields. Their mission was to drop paratroopers in the Gela/ Farello area.

It was expected that during the invasion 15 percent of the men would be sick or wounded. In preparation, burn charts were issued to medical personnel. For example, if both of a man's hands were burned, medical personnel would consult their charts and document that as 4.5 percent of the body; two burned arms equated to 13 percent. Five hundred cc of plasma per each ten percent was given to a burn victim.

The group flew missions daily from North Africa if weather allowed, shuttling troops or supplies to the Sicilian front. On July 30th the group moved to Gabès, across from the island of Djerba off the North African coast.

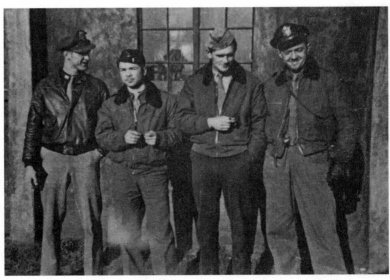

Pilots of the 50th TCS in Sicily

There they practiced glider maneuvers along with other squadrons of the 314th Troop Carrier Group.

Lamb delivered a baby in a fairly well-to-do French home while on Djerba. He was appalled that they didn't keep their house clean. The island of Djerba was filled with dates, figs, olives, almonds, and grapes. Lamb visited a fifteenth-century Spanish fort and enjoyed swimming more than any other activity while he was on the island, but he longed for Tennessee. He thought the French and Arabs were about the filthiest people he had ever seen. Still, his location allowed him the opportunity to visit many new places, including Tripoli, Carthage, Tunis, and Cairo. Lamb also flew over Bethlehem, Jerusalem, and Damascus. He enjoyed the bird's-eye view but was disappointed there were not more landmarks visible from the air.

Men and planes continued to be lost regularly, although most of the fighting on the beach was over after the first week of the invasion. As one pilot said, "Sicily was a land of wrecked planes and bombed-out buildings. There was rubble everywhere." Two weeks after the invasion, Lamb arrived in the Gela area of Sicily and remained there. Before this time, he flew back and forth between Africa and Italy to see to his men. Once he arrived to stay, he set up a dispensary tent and saw to the needs of his men as well as the locals.

On July 16, he wrote home saying he felt rather ashamed of not writing sooner but that he had been very busy lately, as his family must have guessed. The letter was postmarked July 30. Lamb's outfit had played an important part in the invasion of Sicily. His commanding officer received the Distinguished Flying Cross; several of the men had received

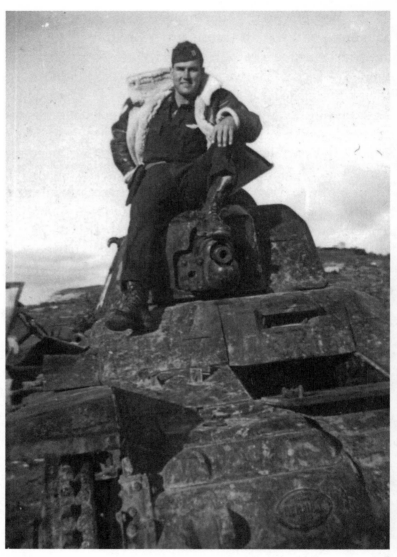

Lamb on top of a French Renault tank near Gela, Sicily

the Air Medal, which was given to crew members who had distinguished themselves meritoriously during an aerial mission. Deserving non-crew members who had flight status that required them to fly regularly were also eligible to receive the award. Lamb did not think the Air Medal meant much, but it had been an experience to receive it. The group was in good spirits and quite confident. Lamb was enjoying good health and weighed 165 pounds. Although it was rough where they were, the men seldom grumbled. Lamb said in his letter, "One doesn't complain when one sees what happens to some of these poor guys. Each day those of us who are alive realize fully how fortunate we are to be alive. Life means a lot when you stop to think of it." Lamb followed with another Letter on July 22 and wrote more about his duties in Sicily:

> In addition to my outfit I have to take care of several hundred British soldiers, as they have no doctors available. They have a great many less doctors than we do. They are nice fellows and very appreciative. Sicily is not much different than North Africa but there are more trees. There are lots of cantaloupes and watermelons. I've eaten a good many of them lately, cause our food is terrible. We occasionally have a good meal. I bought 2 chickens recently and am trying to fatten them up so I can fry them. They are so poor that they don't fatten easily, however.

The IX Troop Carrier Command officially moved on to the new airfield in Sicily on August 10, 1943. The environment in Italy, another hot and arid country, was marginally better than the desert living conditions Lamb had endured in Africa. Cooler than Africa, it had a heavy wind that could blow so hard that the men could hardly talk outside. The

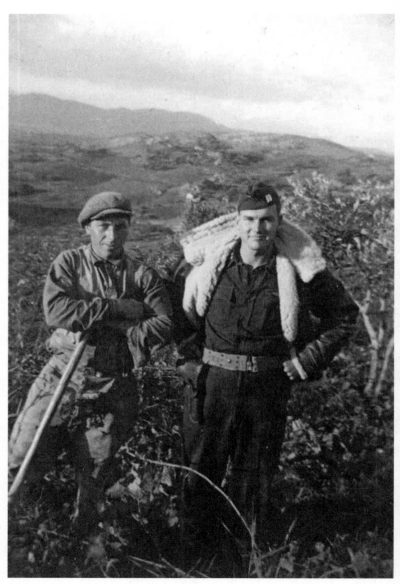

Lamb with a Sicilian farmer

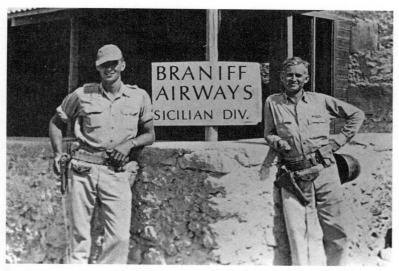

Braniff Airways Sicilian Division. During the war, some of the airline's facilities in the US were used by the military to conduct training exercises for pilots and crewmen.

surrounding land had only small trees and brush, but at least there was some greenery. High mountains, rolling hills, and terraced hillsides overlooking orchards and fields created the landscape. The invasion occurred during the fruit and vegetable season, making tomatoes, peaches, grapes, figs, and mulberries plentiful. Italy was also a country of olive trees, almonds, and chickens.

Buildings were constructed out of the land's native stone, a dull gray, and those structures composed villages that lined the coast. Despite the improved terrain, behind it or in it lay German gun placements well-hidden from the casual view. The roads were horribly dusty and used continuously. Dirt hung in the air. Lamb worked with four medical aides, all of whom reported to him. Before the camp was completed and tents were raised and a clinic established, the group stole an Italian ambulance and used it not only to transport injured but also as living quarters; Lamb and one other man slept in it. So close to the action, Lamb experienced the rapid whine of shelling day and night.

During this time, General Patton's Seventh Army was fighting its way across the northern part of Sicily, pushing the Germans back to Messina. Lamb wrote his family again on August 3, telling them that he had been busy off and on. Recently he had been evacuating wounded out of Sicily by air, what he felt was successful work. "Haven't lost a patient yet in the planes!" he proudly announced. The C-47 had become

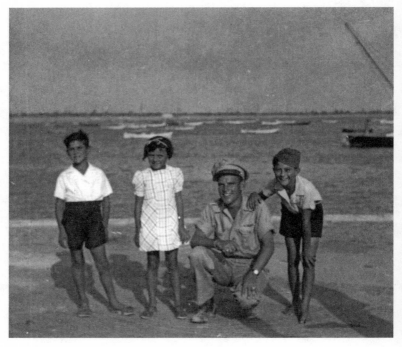

One of the men of the 50th TCS on the Sicilian beach

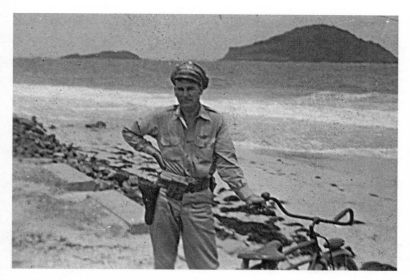

Lamb using a bicycle for transportation around Sicily

an aeromedical workhorse. Most C-47 transports carried an evacuation kit containing blood plasma, oxygen, morphine, portable heaters, first-aid supplies, and various bandages to control hemorrhaging. Lamb went on to write that Patton had recently liberated Palermo. Lamb found Palermo "right pretty" and mentioned it had a big university.

The 314th Troop Carrier Group took over the landing field at Ponte Olivo, a spot just a few miles north of Gela, on August 11, 1943. There were few buildings at that location before the invasion, and after the bombings the pickings were even thinner. The field was a flat area located between the beaches and distant rolling hills. It was an excellent location for an airfield, with one small building situated near the runway. Down time was spent in folding chairs under beech trees writing letters home, talking, listening to the radio, or playing jokes.

Earlier that August, a plane called *Miss Goonie Bird* was badly shot by friendly Navy fire and had barely returned from its mission in one piece. (The name of this specific plane in the 50th TCS was a nod to the nickname of the C-47, "Gooney Bird.") On August 12, *Miss Goonie Bird* crashed at Ponte Olivo. The pilot, Wilbur H. "Buck" Buchanan from Delaware, offered the following account of the event to "Doc" Lamb a number of years later:

> I had a crash once with thirty-two people on board and the plane was a complete disaster and no one was hurt even though the left prop came through the side of the cockpit and cut my pilot's seat back runners off and I went right out through the windshield clear up to the waist not knowing how I got there.
>
> When I saw the fire I pulled myself back through the windshield framework and ran to the rear of the burning aircraft. To my surprise there was no one back there and the cargo of mail was also gone. So I said to myself "I must be in Heaven as I had thirty-two people on this aircraft."
>
> I realized that Jack Schultze [co-pilot] was still in the cockpit so I went back to see why.
>
> "Jack, let's get the hell out of here. This plane is going to blow up."
>
> Jack looked up at me and laughingly said, "Buck, I can't unbuckle my seat belt. I'm hanging on it."
>
> His left leg was stuck through the auto pilot mounting and he was unable to get out. I reached down with my right hand and jerked his safety belt past the built-in arm rest that was holding him, allowing him to get footing and we both walked out of the plane.

Do you remember, Doc, what Joe McClure [commanding officer of the 50th TCS] did right after that crash? He brought me to you after he'd asked me if I felt like flying.

My answer was you bet. Where're we going?

He said, "Hold out your arms, Buck."

I did, and he took hold of both wrists and with a strange look in his eyes said, "For godsake, Buck, you are not even shaking!"

I said, "No, Joe, I'm okay. Where we going?" He said, "Let's go see Doc Myhr to look you over. Then if it's okay we'll go to Africa and get you another airplane."

You shined a light in my eyes and said, "He's okay. His eyes are not even twitching."

So Joe put me in the left seat with two spare pilots in the rear to bring one of the two planes back.

I made two very smooth landings and Joe got out of the plane with me and said, "Buck, I don't believe this. You're okay. Go back to flying tomorrow."[1]

Pilots not only dealt with flying issues while in Sicily but living conditions as well. The heat and lack of sanitation led to diarrhea, malaria, and fevers of unknown origin. The men used mosquito netting, but it did little good. Fleas were also troublesome. Nights were spent fighting bugs, surviving the strafing from German planes, and listening to Allied bombers fly overhead. The Sicilians seemed to be glad the Allies had arrived. Lamb likewise seemed more pleased to be in Europe than he was in Africa; he considered the

Sicilians a harder-working, softer-spoken group of people and much better liked than the lazier Arabs of Africa.

Lamb wrote on August 13 from Sicily that the "gerries blew up lots before they left." He went on to explain that there was still a great deal of shooting going on. Some shots had come close, but so far they had all missed him. Sadly, though, he had lost one of his best friends a few days earlier. His medical practice consisted more of taking care of the nationals than soldiers, he wrote. The people would go around picking up bullets and other stray items. Many came to him because their hands had been blown off after picking up a German anti-personnel mine. The invasion of Sicily was over by August 16, 1943, just a few days after Lamb had written this letter home.

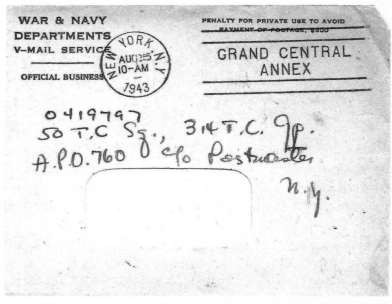

Letter from Lamb sent to his mother by official V-mail, August 1943

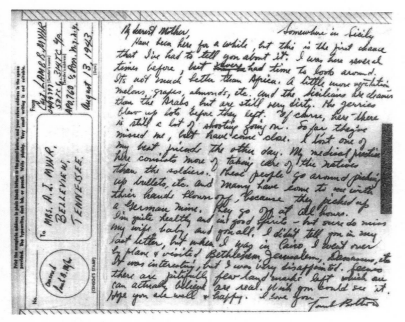

Letter from Lamb sent to his mother by official V-mail, August 1943

On August 19, a medical training program as ordered under the Army Air Forces Memo 25-1 and Medical Training Program Directive No. 1 was established for glider pilots still training in the States. They received twenty-nine hours of first-aid instruction such as tropical disease prevention, desert medicine, treatment of chemical casualties, field sanitation, aviation medicine, and survival and air evacuation of wounded. This was done to prepare pilots in anticipation of the coming invasion of Europe.

On August 21, the 314th Troop Carrier Group left Ponte Olivo for Kairauan in North Africa. However, they returned to Castelvetrano, Sicily, on September 1. By this time the Allied forces controlled the Strait of Messina between Sicily and the mainland of Italy. From this point, the Allies began the move up the boot of Italy.

Almost everything in Italy was made out of rock and stone, and much of it had been pulverized by shelling. Lamb wrote, "I hope those kids [his son and nephews] never have to go thru a mess like this. I'm thankful that our cities will never be bombed and destroyed as these are. I don't see how the people stand it as well as they do."

On September 13, 1943, the group flew a combat mission over Agropoli, Italy. The Allies were securing Naples and working their way towards Rome. Rumors about where the men would be sent next abounded: on into Italy? England? Off to the Pacific? Home?

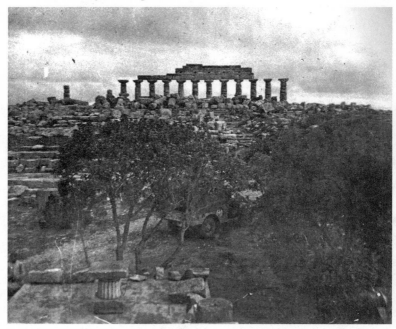

A US Army jeep drives by ruins of a Greek structure in Sicily

Lamb spent two weeks on a small island off the coast of Naples caring for men at a rest camp. He wrote his family a letter early one morning: "You must think I have a lot of spare time, but I do my writing between 5 and 5:20 each morning. It is now a little after 5. Writing takes some time, and helps to take the mind off of unpleasant things. I'm pretty homesick these days."

In Lamb's September 15 letter, he tells of rain so heavy the tents flooded. He began to set his sights on Christmas, writing that it was no longer necessary for his family to send him Milky Ways for the holiday because he could now get them at the Classification Center. He said he looked for gifts to send home, but the Germans had taken almost everything.

That fall, Lamb came down with a case of jaundice and had a difficult time recovering. In his letters, he asked his family for reading material. In order to better communicate, he was learning to read Italian. Lamb could read ten pages of Italian a night and requested that he be sent an Italian/English dictionary. His tent had light, made possible because of a generator. There was less for him to do in Italy than there had been in Africa, but his living conditions were fairly nice. Still, he was tired of being away from home and did not see himself returning before Christmas 1944, more than a year later. He wrote that part of the 314th TCG had already returned to Africa and that the men were pleased with the positive reports out of Russia.

Lamb was not the only one suffering from jaundice during this time; the 50th squadron's monthly report for October stated there had been an epidemic. A visiting epidemiologist from the States interviewed Lamb and the other flight surgeons of the 314th TCG about this and other medical problems their units had been facing. Lamb was relieved of some of his duties while he was sick; for instance, the sex morality lecture, which he would have normally delivered, was given by Chaplain Fowlkes that month.

By that point, Lamb had two tents. He used one for a living room and the other as a bedroom. He also had a small cook stove, enjoyed eating almonds and fresh meat, and looked forward to the oranges ripening in November. While in North Africa he had done his own laundry, in Sicily he paid someone to take over this chore. The men had even built a shower out of old gas tanks. All in all, he thought he was pretty comfortable.

In October 1943, friends and co-workers Lamb, Chaplain Pat Fowlkes, and Dr. Samuel T. Moore, also a flight surgeon, were given some R&R time and decided to take a trip to Naples. Moore summarizes the trip in his book *Flight Surgeon: With the 81st Fighter Group in WWII*:

> Monday, October 25, 1943: Naples
>
> I caught an "early bird" flight to Naples with Captain Lamb Myhr, flight surgeon of the 50th Squadron, and Chaplain Pat Fowlkes of the 314th. . . . A friend of Lamb Myhr met us at the airport with a command car and driver that he put at our disposal. He drove us through the main part of the city to the Parko Hotel on a hill overlooking the harbor. I was somewhat surprised to see very little damage to the city despite reports we had heard of American bombing and German demolition. . . .
>
> Tuesday, October 26, 1943: Naples
>
> Antiaircraft guns started booming at 12:30 a.m. waking

us from a sound sleep. (The battle front is only forty miles north of here.) . . .

We were ordered to evacuate our rooms and take refuge in an air raid shelter carved out of solid rock behind the hotel. My two companions and I dressed quickly . . . One American officer was in such a hurry to get there he didn't take time to dress. He looked pretty ridiculous wearing just his undershorts. . . .

A half hour later the all-clear sounded and we returned to our rooms.

We had breakfast with Major General Terry Allen and Lt. Col. Elliot Roosevelt (FDR's son). Well, sort of . . . they sat at the table next to us.

Business appears to have returned to normal in Naples. (Scarcely three weeks have passed since the city was

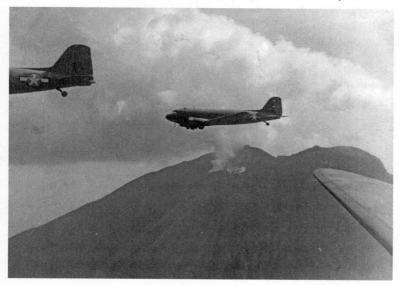

C-47 flying past Mount Vesuvius

liberated.) People scurry here and there as if the war were a thousand miles away. Myhr, [Fowlkes], and I wandered through countless small jewelry, glove, book and variety shops. Prices seemed fairly reasonable. . . .

At noon we returned to the airdrome to catch a 314th transport plane back to our home base. The pilot gave us the grand tour. He completely circled Vesuvius and gave Pompeii a "buzz job."[2]

The eventual inflation of prices in Italy after the trio made this trip was caused by two factors: First, Americans in Italy were willing to pay practically any amount for almost anything. Second, the Italians had no electricity because the Germans had bombed everything before they were driven out of the country. This required items to be made by hand, cutting down on production. From one trip to buy souvenirs to the next, the prices had increased over one hundred percent.

Pat Fowlkes, the chaplain for the 314th group who was on the R&R trip with Lamb, was a close friend. They shared a religious background; Lamb's father had been the secretary of the Christian Church in Tennessee. Also, their particular responsibilities to the men brought them together regularly.

Later that month, Lamb went to Africa to visit the "Vandy Unit." This was the medical unit made up primarily of doctors who had graduated with Lamb from Vanderbilt University medical school. It was not an uncommon occurrence that almost an entire medical unit would be from the same medical school; the same happened with a unit from Harvard, and yet another from the Medical College of Virginia.

In November, Lamb wrote from a rest camp on the Isle Capri. The jaundice epidemic had subsided, and he weighed a healthy 170 pounds. The weather had been quite erratic — it rained sporadically throughout the day and night, which made it difficult to stay warm as his rest-camp tent had no stove. His winter flying clothes came in handy. Morale was fairly high, food was fairly good, and they were happy as long as they were all healthy.

In his letter, Lamb described the island as a beautiful place that would be nice to visit during peace time. While there, he attended the opera in Palermo — he saw *La Traviata* and *The Barber of Seville* — and also heard a fairly good symphonic concert.

He celebrated Thanksgiving on Capri, which included a turkey dinner with all the trimmings. The men were pleased but did not like the thought of going back to spam and corn beef the next day.

Back at Castelvetrano Airfield, where many of the 50th squadron celebrated, "Lights burned late in the 50th kitchen on the night of November twenty-fourth and the festive day dawned bright, crisp, and reasonably clear," recorded the 50th War Dairy. "An autumn tang was in the air, also the inviting aroma of roast turkey. A great day for football, fires in fireplaces, forgiveness of enemies, and feasting." To create some sense of home and holiday tradition, "to round out the afternoon and to perpetuate the American spirit of the day, a football game, of the touch variety, was played, complete with quarters, halves, times out, and semi-officials. The score was in favor of the Officers, they besting the EMs 19-0. All day long the mess hall had visitors, not from squadron personnel, but from fellow squadrons in the Group. Even the Brass graced it with its presence. No inspections, just calling to say 'Hello' . . . They were welcome, of course, but why oh why . . . couldn't they come when 'C' rations were the dish of the day? After all turkey and the fixines' [sic] need time and particular care in preparation."

Later that fall, Lamb revisited Naples, where he tried to buy some gloves. He did not end up purchasing any, as they were only available in odd sizes and the prices had gone up 250 percent since he had last written home. Before he returned to Sicily he went to Malta to see a hospital, which he found to be big, beautiful, and doing excellent work. While there, he found a handkerchief for his mother. In his letters, Lamb continued to write that his friend Pat was always glad to hear of his home state of Virginia. Lamb had family in the state and his sister went to college there, so he often passed on Virginia news from his family's letters to his friend. Lamb was comfortable and healthy, though he was idle most of the time by then. The Allies enjoyed firm control of the island, so there was little fighting.

At the end of the year, Lamb was still in Sicily, and the idleness was bringing him down. He was fed up with lazy Italians, fueled by wine, complaining about their situation. While it was true that the Germans had taken everything from them—and the Allied bombings had destroyed what little they might have had left—"they expect[ed] the Americans and the English to give them everything," Lamb wrote. His background and work ethic led him to believe that they should be working to improve their own situation instead of begging for handouts and taking siestas.

As 1943 came to an end, the 50th squadron reviewed the medical activity of the past months. In the December 1943 report of the squadron medical journal, the team documented some of the highlights:

> There have been a number of unusual happenings in the Squadron this month from a medical standpoint. No new types of diseases have occurred. Only one case of jaundice has been reported in December, and it was a relatively mild case. The venereal disease urethritis has been sulfonamide-resistant, then requiring hospitalization for fever therapy.
>
> In a review of medical data for the past seven months, it is noted that only one member of the Squadron has been returned to the Zone of the Interior for medical reasons. This is a rather remarkable record, as most tactical units usually lose at least 1% of personnel each year from mental disease alone. No combat crew members have been grounded in this Squadron for mental reasons, and there has been no evidence of flying fatigue. Renewal injections of typhoid and typhus vaccines were given to members of the Squadron early in this month.[3]

During the week of November 22-26, President Roosevelt had met with British prime minister Winston Churchill and Chinese president Chiang Kai-shek in Cairo at what became known as the Cairo Conference. There they discussed opening a second front of the war, which would involve the eventual invasion of Normandy.

After the meeting, while he was in that part of the world, Pres. Franklin Roosevelt spent time visiting the troops who had been so successful invading Italy. The invasion had put the Germans on the defensive for the first time in the war.

The significance of the troops' work was not overlooked, and the president's presence giving out medals and shaking hands created a boost in their morale. On December 8, 1943, the commander in chief reviewed the troops of 314th Troop Carrier Group in Sicily. It was a busy, exciting, and important day in the life of the group. The president was pleased with the visit as well, noting later that it was "one of the most successful stopovers" he made.

In attendance were numerous high-ranking Army and Navy officers, including Gen. Henry Harley "Hap" Arnold, head of the Army Air Force; Gen. Dwight D. Eisenhower, the commanding general of the European Theater of Operations; Lt. Gen. Carl Spaatz, commanding general of the Army Air Forces in the European Theater; Lt. Gen. Mark Clark, the commanding general of the Fifth Army; Col. R. H. Tucker, Lt. Col. Joseph B. Crawford, Lt. Lewis H. Brereton, Lt. Edwin F. Gould, and Lt. William C. Kellogg, all members of the Fifth Army; Lt. Gen. George S. Patton, Jr., of the Seventh Army; Maj. Gen. James J. Doolittle, Special Air Force; Maj. Gen. W. B. Smith, chief of staff of the North African Theater of Operations; Brig. Gen. Paul L. Williams, commanding general of the IX Troop Carrier Command; Brig. Gen. H. L. Clark, commanding general of the 52nd Troop Carrier Wing; Brig. Gen. Frank McSherry, head of the Allied Military Government Office; Harry L. Hopkins, personal advisor to the president; Maj. Gen. Edwin M. Watson, military aide to the president; Adm. William Leahy, the president's special advisor on military and naval affairs; Rear Adm. Ross T. McIntire, personal physician to the president; and officers of the Allied Military Government for Occupied Territories who were currently in Italy.

President Roosevelt awarded the Distinguished Service Cross to Mark Clark, Tucker, Crawford, Kellogg, Brereton, and Gould of the Fifth Army that day. Since Lamb had a camera, General Clark instrùcted him to take pictures of the event. However, Lamb's commanding officer gave him an ever more interesting duty — to monitor President Roosevelt's liquor. A plane was en route from Cairo specifically for the purpose of delivering the president's Scotch. "Doc, if they want a drink of whiskey you give them yours if the other doesn't get here in time," Lamb was told. As a security measure, he was also instructed to act as bartender, thereby ensuring that Eisenhower and the other dignitaries would not be poisoned. It was a significant

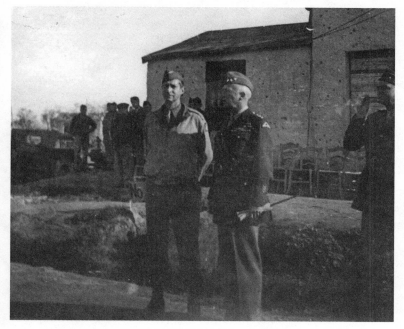

Gens. Mark Clark and George Patton

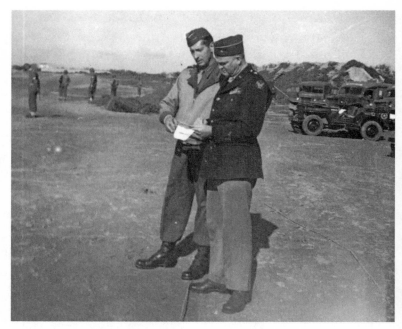

Gen. Mark Clark and a fellow US general

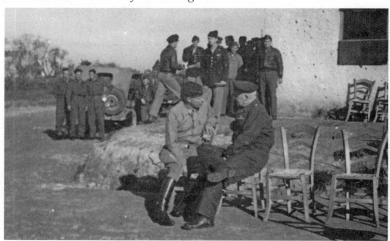

General Eisenhower (right) *conversing with a fellow US general*

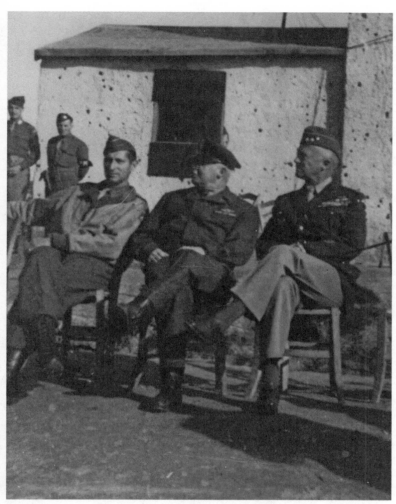

Gens. Clark, Eisenhower, and Patton

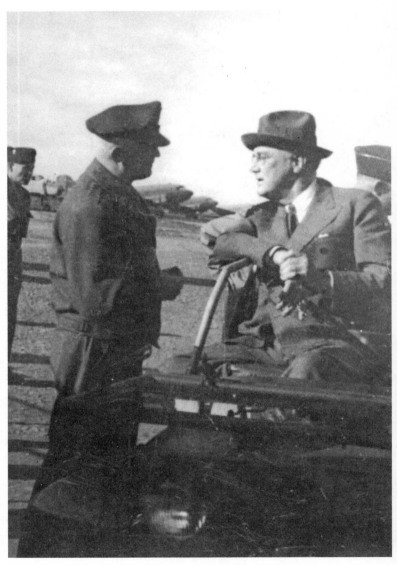

General Eisenhower speaking with President Roosevelt

assignment, one that showed the commanding officer trusted Lamb.

US Gens. Hap Arnold, Mark Clark, and George Patton, who were present during the president's visit to the 314th Troop Carrier Group, met in Sicily to discuss the invasion of Italy. Generals Clark, who would command the movement north, and Patton, whose success in North Africa was well-known, were both graduates of the United States Military Academy at West Point.

Lamb's squadron, the 50th Troop Carrier Squadron, won the Presidential Unit Citation for their work during the invasion of Sicily. The Army Presidential Unit Citation, in ribbon form, was awarded to units for heroic actions against an armed enemy during hazardous conditions. Gen. Matthew Ridgway, who commanded the paratroopers of the 82nd Airborne, was unable to account for forty-three of his paratroopers, but the division was honored nonetheless; Patton stated the airborne had saved the assault forty-eight additional hours. Troop carriers and paratroopers had been an instrumental force in the war so far. Lessons learned during the fighting in North Africa and Italy would prove invaluable in the preparation for the invasion of Normandy. Lamb's squadron was rumored to be stationed in England next; though that assignment had not yet been verified, the men were already looking forward to the positive living conditions in that country.

One of Lamb's additional duties was to participate in special court-martials as defense counsel. All flight surgeons were required to take their turn in this position when a case came up. Lamb was appointed to this role in December;

he was to evaluate the defendant and give his professional opinion on the man's mental soundness.

For Lamb, Christmas 1943 was spent watching the 2nd Annual "Holiday Harmonies" Christmas presentation. Officers and enlisted of the 50th TCS attended. There was a nineteen-member choral group, and twelve men preformed skits. The program required an eight-man technical staff to run smoothly. Afterward, everyone enjoyed a turkey dinner.

On December 27, Lamb wrote to his mother back in Tennessee about the Christmas holiday and recent events:

> My dearest mother,
>
> Thanks so much for making this a nice Christmas for me. The cake was excellent, and I appreciate the trouble you had to find the ingredients these days. All who tasted the cake [were] very complimentary. You make them just as good as you did in those days when I would eat most of the nuts before you could put them in the cake.
>
> The Mediterranean winters were damp and cold, but rarely below freezing. I have a stove in my tent and spend most of my time reading. Please don't send me any more papers because I needed to travel light, and don't want to accumulate any more than necessary.
>
> Also thanks for the excellent picture. Pat Fowlkes and others were very impressed with the handsomeness of my family. Especially there [were] some extremely nice remarks about Lene, whom several thought was very pretty. They thought she looked rather glamorous also with that lock of hair down over one eye. Betty sent two nice photos the other day which really made me quite happy. The boy is growing so fast. Yes, I had hoped to be there when he started walking and talking but I suppose I'll have to wait and see the next one go thru those stages.

The President and all the 4-star generals were here recently to visit our field. They stayed a couple of hours. We had a parade and the normal stuff that goes with all that. The President looked well and rather confident. We have utmost confidence in General Eisenhower. Thanks again for the nice presents. One of my new years' resolutions is to write you more often.

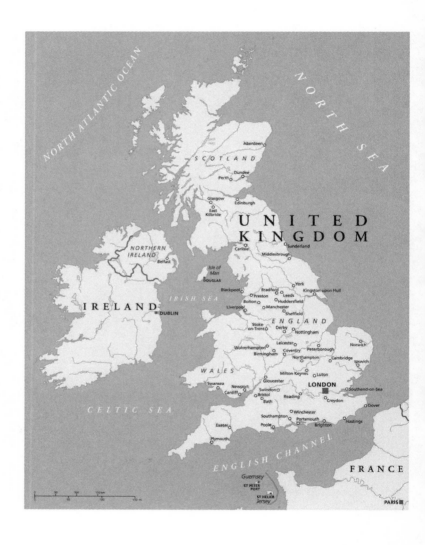

Chapter Five
England

In February 1944, Lamb was transferred to the United Kingdom to prepare for the invasion of Germany. On February 16, the air echelon moved to Castelvetrano, Sicily, to organize for the relocation. The ground echelon would depart from Palermo, Sicily. One quarter of the IX Troop Carrier Command was transferred to Italy to help Patton with the invasion of southern France before the rest left Sicily.

Lamb was part of the advance party. His movement orders were posted on February 12th and documented by the following notation in the 50th War Diary:

Capt. Lamb B. Myhr, Serial number 0419797

Left Feb 15 from Castelvetrano, Sicily to the United Kingdom for permanent change of station.

Orders were issued for the men not to take cotton clothing with them. They were leaving their light attire behind for wool clothes needed in the cold, damp English winter weather.

The Ninth Air Force moved in waves. The designations were A, B, C, D, and E. The 50th squadron was slated for the C wave. Each man was issued five days of either C or K rations. The following embarkation uniform and equipment was ordered for each officer and enlisted man: O.D. (Officer of the Day) overcoat, O.D. shirt and pants, G.I. shoes and leggings, full field equipment and helmet (field jacket rolled in field bag), gas mask, raincoat, weapon, and horseshoe blanket rolled and slung over left shoulder containing: shelter half, line pole and pins, three blankets, and fatigue suit.

Consisting of ten planes, the advance echelon, which included Lamb, left for England on February 12. The planes stopped at Tunis to refuel, where they were then delayed for three days because of poor weather. Housing was available, making the layover comfortable. When the advance echelon took off again, they flew to Oran, Algeria, the best place to stop before nightfall; because their lights could be seen by the enemy, the planes did not fly in the dark. Adequate lodging was again secured so men didn't have to sleep on the ground or in the plane. On February 16, the echelon of ten planes was continuing its journey and flying over Marrakech when the weather turned bad again, causing ice to accumulate on the wings of the planes. They were instructed to return to base at Oran. However, two aircraft could not be reached by radio. While the remaining planes, one of which included Lamb, returned to Oran, these two continued their flight and arrived in England in approximately twelve hours. The other eight planes arrived at Saltby Airfield in Leicestershire, England, on February 20.

The air echelon had flown along the coast of Africa in a complicated dogleg route in order to avoid German naval guns and not fly over any German-controlled territory. Being within reach of land-based German planes made those taking the 1,680-mile trip nervous.

In Palermo, the ground echelon boarded the troopship *Monarch of Bermuda* on March 5. They had air cover and strong surface support the entire trip. During peace time, the *Monarch of Bermuda*, a British cruise ship, made leisure trips between New York and Bermuda. On March 19, the echelon made port in Greenock, Scotland, and arrived at Station 538 the following day. The IX AFSC (Air Force Service Command) Intransit Depot Group handled all the logistics of moving, including transporting supplies and planes from place to place. They would continue the same services after the invasion of France and took on the additional responsibility of transferring the wounded.

The incessant cold, windswept, foggy weather of middle Britain was an abrupt change from the arid climate Lamb had experienced in Sicily. To alleviate combat exhaustion, a rotation of leave was established, giving men a week off after

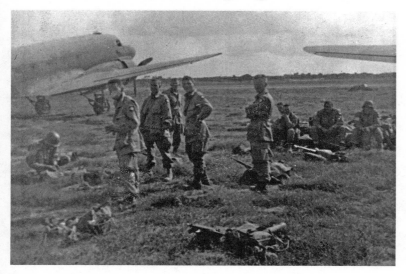

Paratroopers waiting to load for a mission from England

arriving at their new station. Americans, including Lamb, found it difficult to find their way around because signposts and directional signs had been removed in anticipation of a German invasion.

Lamb had become part of the military operation code-named Bolero, which was the influx of men and supplies into Britain. Southern England soon became one gigantic armed camp in preparation for the invasion of Normandy, code-named Roundup. Veterans of the North Africa and Sicily campaigns had been brought to England to teach replacements how to prepare for the upcoming offensive.

Lamb, along with the rest of the IX Troop Carrier Command, 52nd Troop Carrier Wing, 314th Troop Carrier Group, 50th Troop Carrier Squadron, was posted at Station 538 at Saltby. The command was located eleven miles south of Grantham and fifty miles north of London in the English Midlands. Grantham was a quiet town where not much happened to interest the visiting soldiers. Nottingham was the largest city in the area. The men enjoyed some of their off time in town at a pub called the Robin Hood Inn.

The IX Troop Carrier Command (TCC) came under the leadership of Brig. Gen. Paul L. Williams after their arrival in England. Born in Detroit, Williams had extensive training as a pilot. Before taking over the Ninth US Army Air Force, he served in the Eighth US Army Air Force in England, helping to plan the strategic bombing of German industries. Because of his contributions during the war, he was later considered a great air tactician.

The fields were given letters for code purposes. Lamb's new station was called Field J. It consisted of three country roads that were used as grass airstrips. The airfield was, quite literally, a cow pasture. When the field originally opened in August 1941, Group 92 of the British Royal Air Force Bomber Command used it as a satellite field. It was overlaid with chicken wire, and after one week of heavy pounding from the 50th TCS's C-47s taking off and landing, the runways were reduced to nothing more than extremely hazardous ruts and bumps.

IX TCC units used three main field centers. The first included fields in Lincolnshire and one each in the adjacent countries of Rutland and Northamptonshire. The second center was made up of four inland fields in Berkshire and one in Wiltshire, while the third was near the coast of the English Channel with two fields in Devon and two in Somerset. The IX Army Air Forces Troop Carrier Command

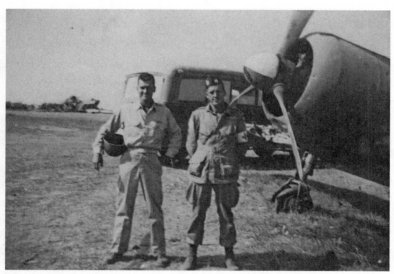

Lamb (left) and an aide in front of a C-47 and ambulance on the airfield

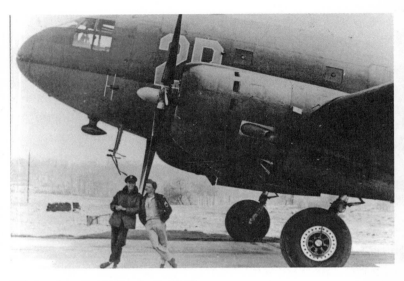

Pilot and copilot in front of a C-47

Headquarters was located in St. Vincents Hall in Grantham.

The Ninth Army Air Force joined the Eighth Army Air Force in December 1943 as part of the Allied Expeditionary Air Force, a segment of the First Allied Airborne Army. The Ninth was flexible between RAF and US Army Air Forces, and the commanding officers of the Airborne Divisions were used as needed by either command. When the Ninth Air Force arrived in England, additional bomber groups, fighter groups, and troop carrier groups were added and leadership was reorganized. Thus, when the IX Troop Carrier Command arrived at their new station in England, they were a part of an almost entirely new Ninth Air Force. Chain of command was formed into wings that each controlled three to five groups. Each group was in turn made up of three or four squadrons and had its own field.

More than two hundred planes per wing were preparing to fly to Normandy.

Fields were supposed to be located beyond the effective range of German bombers, but Lamb's station did experience some damage. Before the landing fields could be used again, wreckage had to be cleared and holes repaired. German V-1 flying bombs, also known as buzz bombs, continued to fly over the fields. The station was bombed three additional times by the Luftwaffe while Lamb was in the area. Luckily, there was little damage during these raids.

The 121st Station Hospital at Braintree was not so fortunate. A successful German bombing demolished nine wards, completely flattening two. Though many of the wards were filled with patients, the bombing caused only minor injuries.

When the men of the 50th squadron arrived in England, their initial reaction to the base at Saltby was that it was immense; they admired its concrete runways, ample taxiways, parking and hangers for aircraft, Officers' Club, Enlisted Men's Club, Officers' Mess, and Enlisted Men's Mess. One soldier remarked that "they were being treated like first class soldiers." The command had gone from the slums to uptown living.

On the new base, superior officers were saluted, whereas protocol had been much more relaxed in Africa and Italy. Officers and enlisted men did not cross established military lines. Administrative duties were tightened—there were no excuses for late reports—and gas mask drills became a regular occurrence. The field and planes were guarded well. Blackout conditions continued each night.

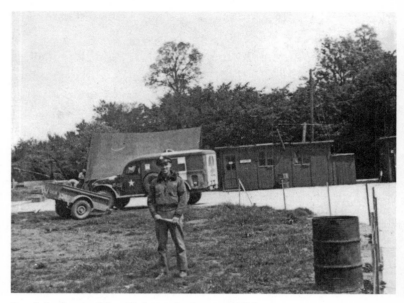

Lamb in front of the clinic on the base at Saltby

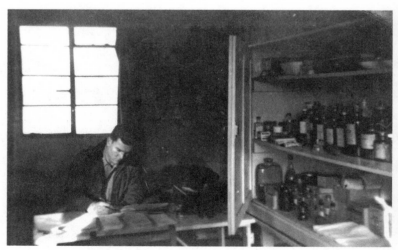

Lamb filling out paperwork in the dispensary

Dress uniforms were worn and cleaned regularly, which had not been the case in a long time. Uniforms were mandatory at supper, whether it was eaten in the Officers' Mess or in town. The men were required to wear neckties and dress shirts at all official events as well as at the Officers' Club and at monthly dances, for which local ladies were brought in to attend. The clubs were well stocked with liquor. At the Officers' Mess, white tablecloths were used.

Each of the men was given a "Guide to Britain" that provided advice on living in England. The guide suggested not to throw money around, not to boast about being there to save England, and not to underestimate British fortitude. It was apparent to Lamb that the English had suffered much during the last three years.

Many of the men were billeted in Nissen huts, which were models for American Quonset huts. Similar in construction,

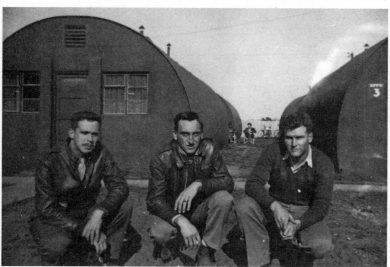

Lamb (right) and two pilots in front of the barracks

both the Nissen and Quonset huts consisted of curved corrugated sheet metal with bricked ends and featured windows on either side of a door at each end of the structure. The concrete floors made for dry living conditions, which were greatly appreciated in the rainy English weather.

A nearby central latrine served several huts. The latrine included a washroom with running water all the time and hot water in the mornings. Hot showers were available on Saturdays; schedules were posted allowing twenty minutes per man. The downside was that none of the buildings were insulated. Because of the high humidity and dampness and the generally low temperatures, the buildings were cold. Without insulation, the temperature indoors was usually the same as the outdoor temperature. Each hut contained a small Sibley stove made out of thin sheet metal bent into a cone shape. This type of stove was originally intended for a tent. While it was useful for warming hands, it did not give off enough heat to warm the hut.

Despite the chill, Lamb found his hut much more accommodating than the tent or ambulance he had called home in Africa. Months had passed since he had slept inside a building, had a real bed, and could count on a warm shower regularly. He was glad to be in a civilized country again, away from the heat and dirt of Africa.

Still, the winter proved a harsh, challenging one for the men stationed in England. Fuel shortages plagued enlisted men and officers alike. Unable to count on the military's supply of fuel, coal, and stoves to keep warm, men took to cutting down trees and scavenging for any other heat source they could find. In these conditions, flight surgeons were often called on to "parent" the pilots, helping them manage and adjust to their new surroundings. Flight surgeon Lt. Col. Ernest Galliard, Jr., of the Eighth Air Force provided such a report of an English camp:

> Another thing that has come to my attention about the fuel shortage is that such notables as Capt. Murray, the ex-professor of anatomy, and Capt. Bland, Flight Surgeon of the 535th BS, have been visiting the ash piles behind the enlisted men's barracks and are quite enthusiastic about the "big pieces" of coke [coal] they had salvaged. Some ingenious members of the organization have found that a six pence can of shoe polish is a good substitute for kindling wood and that the shoe impregnate is supposed to protect against noxious gases is also a highly inflammable item.
>
> Praise the Lord! At last we have found a useful use for this material we have been toting across the world for the past six months.[1]

The men adjusted quickly to living and working in what

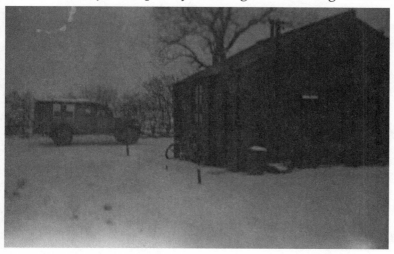

Snow covering the camp during a cold English winter

would still be considered primitive conditions. They were quite innovative in making themselves comfortable: They cut trees to make clothes racks, twisted bits of wire into clothes hangers, and fashioned scavenged metal into a cooking grill to boil water for washing. Lamb described his new accommodations in a letter to his mother:

> I like England in comparison to other places overseas. I have been living in a wooden barracks and have a room with a small stove. Coal is rationed. The food is better here and we have butter occasionally. English climate is terrible. It is so dark and dreary throughout the day and quite cold early in the morning. We have had a good snow here recently, but it has melted today.
>
> God bless you and keep you always, your son,

When the pilots were not flying, they loafed, wrote letters, played cards, or just talked. To the great joy of Lamb and all the other men, the mail arrived regularly. They craved any news from the US, and sharing letters became a ritual. Lamb requested that his sister send him the addresses of family members living in England but instructed her to make no comment about their relationship to him. Should the letters fall into enemy hands and the Axis Powers learn of the relation, Lamb's family in Europe could be in danger. Lamb enjoyed his R&R more in England than he had in Africa because he spoke the language. He spent his weekly time off in town. Lamb was able to make a trip to London while he was stationed in the country, which he wrote his family about on March 12, 1944:

> Have just come back from London, where I visited for a

few days. Saw many of the things I had wondered about.
I guess things have changed quite a bit there, because the
place is different from the way I had pictured it. It is quite
an expensive place, so I doubt if I'll go there again anytime
soon. I saw some of the legendary places and also saw a few
good plays, one by Charles Corgene with John Gilgood.

Love to everyone,

In his book *Brave Men,* Ernie Pyle shared his impressions
of Army Air Force life in a station similar to Lamb's:

I almost never heard an airman griping about things
around there.

It was an old station, and well established. Our men were
comfortably housed and wonderfully fed. The officers had
a club of their own, with a bar and a lounge room, and the
Red Cross provided a big club right on the station for the
enlisted men.

There were all kinds of outdoor games, such as baseball,
badminton, volleyball, tennis and even golf at a nearby
town. One of the pilots came back from golfing and said,
"I don't know what they charged me a greens fee for, I was
never anywhere near the greens."

At first I lived with the younger officers of the squadron,
then I moved over with the enlisted gunners, radiomen, and
flight engineers. They lived only a little differently. And the
line between officer and enlisted men among the combat
crews was so fine that I was barely aware of any difference
after a few days' acquaintance with them.

First I'll try to tell you how the officers lived. I stayed in
the hut of my friends Lieutenants Lindsey Greene and Jack
Arnold. There was usually a spare cot in any hut, for there
was almost always one man away on leave. Their barracks

was a curved steel Nissen hut, with doors and windows at each end but none along the sides. The floor was bare concrete. Eight men lived in the hut. Three were pilots, the other bombardiers and navigators. One was a captain, the others were lieutenants.

The boys slept on black steel cots with cheap mattresses. They had rough white sheets and Army blankets. They were all wearing summer underwear then, and they slept in it. When the last one went to bed he turned out the light and opened one door for ventilation. Of course until the lights were out the hut had to be blacked out.

Each cot had a bed lamp rigged over it, with a shade made from an empty fruit-juice can. The boys had a few bureaus and tables they bought or dug up from somewhere. On the tables were pictures of their girls and parents, and on the corrugated steel walls they had pasted pin-up girls from Yank and other magazines.

In the center of the hut was a rectangular stove made of two steel boxes welded together. They burned wood or coal in it, and it threw out terrific heat. In front of the stove was a settee big enough for three people and behind the stove was a deep chair. Both settee and chair were made by nailing small tree limbs together. The boys did it themselves.

In the top of the hut, when the lights went out, I could see two holes with moonlight streaming through. Somebody shot his .45 one night, just out of exuberance. Somebody else then bet he could put a bullet right through that hole. He lost his bet, which accounted for the other hole.

The latrines and washbasins were in a separate building about fifty yards from the hut. The boys and their mechanics had built a small shower room out of packing boxes and rigged up a tank for heating water. They were proud of it, and they took plenty of baths.

All around my hut were similar ones, connected by concrete or cinder paths. The one next door was about the fanciest. Its name was Piccadilly Place, and it had a pretty sign over the door saying so. In the hut the boys had built a real brick fireplace, with a mantel and everything.

In there the biggest poker game was usually going. A sign on the front of the hut said, "Poker Seats by Reservation Only." On the other side of the door was another sign saying, "Robin Hood Slept Here." They put that up when they first arrived because somebody told them the station was in Sherwood Forest. They found out later they were a long way from Sherwood Forest but they left the sign up anyhow.

It was a good station. The boys were warm, clean, well fed, their life was dangerous and not very romantic to them, and between missions they got homesick and sometimes bored. But even so they had a pretty good time with their live young spirits and they were grateful that they could live as well and have as much pleasure as they did have. For they knew that anything good in wartime is just that much velvet.[2]

As nice as the men thought the living conditions were in England, there were many complaints about English-prepared food. Powdered eggs, fried Spam, brussels sprouts, and creamed chicken on toast were the usual fare. Most of the men hated English coffee and found the tea too strong. There was a lack of milk and very little butter available. Many thought the mutton was the worst. The scent of it cooking permeated the camp for hours before it was served. Some of the men preferred to catch rabbit for their meals. Actually, the Army Air Forces were abundantly supplied, and the IX Troop Carrier Command lived well.

Camps were moved regularly and men were relocated

between camps. This provided them with valuable experience for the Normandy invasion, when they were moved between units while on the continent. Mobility exercises coincided with the base movements. Groups not scheduled for an immediate change of station were directed to carry out such exercises by leap-frogging between the adjacent countryside and back again. Sometimes the transportation for these moves was not available, so imaginary or simulated trucks were staked out in a spot to represent a conveyance. Each individual was responsible for finding his own way to his next camp if there was no transportation provided.

In some cases, the mobility exercises involved the movement of all available personnel and materials and their re-establishment in readiness for operations. Closer to invasion time, some groups moved to the London area from the Midlands to be closer to the coast.

Chapter Six
Keeping Them Flying

Upon arrival at a new camp, Lamb's first duty was to establish station sick quarters. Using this small hospital, his chief job was to "keep the pilots flying." Lamb handled general medical care while he was stationed in Grantham, from February to July 1944.

Squadron medical detachments were joined to form one large detachment that cared for all personnel at the station. Sick quarters was located away from the flight line but close enough that evacuation was available. The building had two wards (one for officers and one for enlisted men), a crash room for emergency surgical procedures, a sick call room, a pharmacy, a medical supply store room, a small laboratory, and offices for Lamb and the other flight surgeons. There was also a room for the administrative branch of the detachment. A decontamination center beside these quarters was arranged the same way and had the same facilities. The dental department was set up in other quarters in an area close by. In those same quarters was also a ward for overflow patients from the station sick quarters that was used to tend to patients with venereal disease and other contagious diseases.

A small Army Air Force hospital was staffed by at least

two doctors, a dentist, and about fifteen medics. Despite the general shortage of medical personnel during the war, the IX TCC enjoyed a full staff of flight surgeons and medics in their hospitals while they were stationed in England. There were forty aviation medical dispensaries or small hospitals activated to support the months of preparation before the Normandy invasion and the needs of the men after the offensive. Around 8,300 doctors and 3,700 nurses were stationed in England during the spring of 1944. A pilot gave this account of the medical work done in his squadron during that time:

> One section that functioned smoothly—perhaps in part because it had responsibilities that were almost too easy for its personnel—the medical unit. The Squadron Flight surgeon had a long list of responsibilities in addition to being what today would be our primary care physician. He supervised our immunization shots and booster; cared for the injuries our Engineering people suffered on the line; made sure all our medical records were up to date; checked on our water supply and sanitary facilities (Latrines); tried to guard against venereal disease; and decided when one of us had to be hospitalized. But he had three medical assistants, one of who [sic] was qualified as a medical technician and the other as a surgical technician.[1]

Flight surgeons were also supported by medics, who made sure the first aid kits in each airplane and glider were complete and in good shape. In addition, medics helped facilitate the routine known as sick call. Men would come to the dispensary first thing in the morning after reveille with their complaints or for the occasional and always-unannounced venereal disease inspection.

While in England, VD tended to be the widest-spread

medical problem. The Air Surgeon's Office issued numerous directives regarding the disease; when penicillin became plentiful in late 1944, shots were issued once a week to suppress any outbreak. In addition, each man received one sulfa tablet with breakfast every day. With one hundred men in the squadron's engineering section alone, this was a time-consuming job. With the influx of men, Lamb had to be continually supplied with serum for shots. The non-commissioned officer helping Lamb gave most of the injections under the doctor's guidance.

On March 7, the 39th Field Hospital was officially assigned to the Ninth Air Force. Back in December 1943, the 810th Medical Air Evacuation Squadron had also been assigned to the command. They were given the job of evacuating hospitalized American military personnel from Ireland to England. Two planes flew as part of the evacuation squadron from Maghaberry, Ireland, to Pershore, England, constituting the command's first genuine operational mission. It was required that a registered nurse be assigned to each medical evacuation flight; Lamb and his medics participated in only a few of these evacuations. From Pershore, the injured men were loaded on a ship to return to the States. Flights such as these became a regular feature of the Troop Carrier Command's operations.

All in all, Lamb's hospital work in England was less demanding than it had been in Africa or Sicily. He wrote his mother about this on March 31, 1944:

Dearest Mother,

Guess you've wondered why I have written so little lately. The main reason is that there is so very little to write about. I received your letter of March 17 today and was glad to hear that you are well. Not much is happening here. I have found Bill Freeland's [Lamb's brother-in-law] location and will probably look him up in a few days. We have set up a small hospital here on our base, and it is enjoyable to be doing a little hospital work again, even tho' it is very little. I plan to do some traveling in England if I am able to get some time off. We are occasionally allowed 48 hrs passes. I spent several days in London and saw some good plays while there.

The weather is rather cold here, and of course the coal shortage is rather extreme now that the Welch miners are on strike. We are having snow occasionally, but on the whole, the spring weather in England is not too bad. I have a small stove in my room which I am allowed to start after 5PM, so I'm comfortable enough.

Glad you received the candy. Wish I could have sent you something better. Take care of yourself.

I miss you honey and think of you every day and night.

Take care of yourself,

Regular medical staff meetings were held at the station hospital. The medical detachment of the 314th TCG operated as a pseudo-independent organization. It had its own living area for the enlisted men made up of two barracks that sat adjacent to the main sick quarter's installation. An acting detachment commander was appointed through whom the enlisted men received their duty assignments, passes, and supplies. This commander was also the individual these men went to if they had any issues with their patients.

All flight surgeons handled daily sick call and ward

duties regardless of other assignments. Charge of the wards rotated by the week, and MOD (medical officer of the day) duties were alternated daily. When missions were scheduled, two flight surgeons attended each briefing and saw the planes off. The medical department issued candy rations to every member of the crew leaving on a mission in order to keep up the crew member's energy. Coffee and cookies were also offered before takeoff by the ambulance drivers and medics.

On the planes' return from a mission, five ambulances were stationed by the control tower and at the head of the runway to receive casualties. At least two medical officers were present. In addition to the regular first-aid kits, they had a surgical kit available for emergency treatment.

The base medical service was divided into different sections with an officer in charge of each. These duties would rotate. For example, Lamb might be designated as equipment liaison officer for a time. In this role, he would serve as a liaison between the medical department and the group equipment office. His responsibility was to know the status of the equipment at all times and keep a close check on the various first-aid kits on the aircraft. Another officer would be assigned the duty of the base medical inspector, responsible for venereal-disease and respiratory-disease control and other disease-related issues.

Lamb's April 1944 medical report indicated that the upper respiratory issues had increased in camp. There was one case of meningitis, but there were fewer cases of VD than ever recorded in the previous theater. The next month, Lamb's entry into the 50th War Dairy Squadron Medical

Journal specified that this positive trend continued in May:

> The usual number of cases of upper respiratory infections has been reported this month. The damp English weather has been a causative factor in increasing the number of cases of sinusitis. However, in spite of this, the number of actual days lost among flying personal [sic] has been relatively small in comparison to previous months.
>
> There have been no venereal diseases reported this month. This is rather remarkable as it is the second successive month in which none have been reported. There is no obvious explanation for this remarkable phenomenon.
>
> In general, the health of the squadron personal [sic] has been good. There have been no epidemics of communicable disease. One death occurred, that being a self-inflicted gunshot as the result of an anxiety neuroses.
>
> Lamb B. Myhr
>
> Capt, MC.[2]

The upper echelon medical officer made regular visits to review decisions of sanitation, water cleanliness, and living conditions. The flight-surgeon-designated inspector usually made his rounds on Saturdays unless they were needed more often. Maj. Gen. David N. W. Grant, the first air surgeon of the Army Air Forces (1941-1945), understood how important these regular rounds were to maintaining the health of the men in the Army Air Forces. As he stated, "personal care does not end with the squadron Flight Surgeon . . . [T]o assure the maintenance of the striking force of the air command medical service must include hospital, sanitary, and daily hygiene inspection of facilities."[3]

Such inspections were made throughout the commands of the Army Air Forces, including within the 50th Troop Carrier Squadron. They were often documented in the war dairy similarly to this entry from July 1943:

July 6 Thorough investigation of food problem at the Consolidated Mess for the noon meal was investigated. The meal consisted of Beef and Vegetable Stew, which had carrots and no evidence of spoilage existed; string beans, also canned, spinach and potatoes, steam cooked. There seemed to be a rumor of an addition of a small quantity of sausage (canned Vienna style) which were added at the last minute. The sausage was supposed to have been previously opened, whether this is actually the case, and when the can was actually opened is a problem to which no satisfactory answer is available.

July 7 All patients have come through their trouble in good shape except for two cases who seemed pretty well exhausted, there were complicating factors. No history of other possibilities regarding the food problem exists. Possibilities of dirty mess kits or faulty washing have been considered, also possibility of dirty containers used in serving food. No conclusions have been deduced, as the facts do not seem to bear out any single possibility or clue.

It has been decided to make entries of early sanitary inspections, whether of any scope or not, to have some idea of the condition of various places over a period of time. So little is being done to remedy the situation it is pitiful.

Site #6. Enlisted combat crew site ablutions is very dirty. Paper and dirt are littered over the floor, toilets have not been scrubbed and no basins are present for washing. There is no hot water because no coal is available. Some coal shortage exists, and it seems that coal for heating water was removed by personnel living on the site for heating huts.

Fuel sufficient for heating huts is not available at this time. Explanation for dirty conditions of huts and ablutions is that brooms, brushes, etc., are not available.

Site #3. Washroom has no hot water for same reason as above.

Site #7. Has no hot water as the containers have not been set up.

Communal Site. The bath house has very little hot water. Temperature of water was 80 degrees. Many of the showers are leaky, and it is presumed that much of the hot water leaks out as large quantities are being used. Showers are dirty and have not been scrubbed satisfactorily at any time.[4]

Vomiting and diarrhea from possible food poisoning caused by poor food preparation was common. These incidences could be so severe that up to twenty-five or thirty men would be admitted to the hospital at one time for nausea, vomiting, and diarrhea.

If there was a breakout of an illnesses like cholera, typhus, tetanus, or other infectious disease, or if there were a number of causalities, Lamb was extremely busy. Until early 1944, most of the military hospitals were located in southern England, while most air stations were located in northern England. The small base hospital was the first line of defense against health problems for many months.

Lamb had exchanged the medical issues of the dry desert for those of the chill, constantly damp English climate. Many men found the English winter insufferably cold, the rain freezing, and the accompanying inches of deep mud difficult. Since mud was always most considerable during the rainy, snowy English winters, it reminded the men of winter year-round, no matter the season. The American soldiers had no waterproof boots, which contributed to frostbite and trench foot. Heated gloves, boots, heavy socks, and glove liners were in short supply. Frostbite was a particularly persistent issue because the pilots regularly flew at high altitudes. Even in July and August, it remained a problem.

Ruptured appendices, kidney stones, and minor cuts and abrasions were common, some of which occurred while the men were cutting wood for fuel or looking for coal. Injuries from motorcycle accidents, car accidents, and kitchen mishaps were also among those treated by Lamb regularly. Bicycle accidents were responsible for many minor injuries, but occasionally crash-related wounds were serious enough to hospitalize a man for several weeks. One flight surgeon noted in a hospital report that "the frequency of [bicycle] accidents is increasing almost beyond reason." Lamb often tended to fractured legs, which required splinting. Gangrene was a serious threat, but with the availability of penicillin Lamb was fortunately able to save most men's limbs.

Amidst the unavoidable injuries associated with war, Lamb also witnessed an inane number of senseless accidents. In one case, a truck and a jeep collided head-on, causing head injuries to the drivers. In June of 1944, a sergeant in the 7th Station Complement Squadron was accidentally — but fatally — shot by a friend with a Thompson submachine gun in the barracks.

Of course, there was no shortage of war-related wounds

to see to. These included injuries from German fire bombs, or incendiary bombs, and plane crashes during landing.

One accident on the flight line of a bomber group occurred during the process of loading three-hundred pound bombs on a B-17. Two explosions within fifteen to thirty seconds of one another were followed by a blazing fire. Twenty-two enlisted men and one officer were killed instantly, and a British civilian who was cycling past the site was fatally wounded, dying a few minutes after arriving at station sick quarters. Injuries included a contaminated compound leg fracture, blast injuries to the chest, sprained ankles, and minor abrasions. Ten soldiers who were present at the time were not positively accounted for after the incident; the bodies and mutilated remains of thirteen men were collected, but these were too charred and disfigured to identify.[5]

Frequently after a mission, flak had to be removed from crew members. One flight surgeon recalled a pilot he treated who had a small wad of flak in his shoulder. The pilot was not concerned about his wound; instead, he complained loudly about not being fed before the shell fragment was removed. In January 1944, a flak suit became standard equipment available to every crew member, an addition that resulted in fewer injuries and deaths from flak and cannon fire. (At around the same time, improvements were made to flight helmets as well.) The Wilkinson Sword company produced the armored suit, which they called a flak vest. Made of thin manganese plates positioned to protect the chest and pelvic area, a vest weighed around twenty-five pounds.

After suffering a severe injury during a mission, a gunner reflected on the value of his flak suit in the following statement:

I'm getting the Purple Heart for my wound. If it weren't for the flak suit, I'd be getting the Purple Heart posthumously. The bullet, a .30 cal, went through the suit, knocking one of the pieces out. It careened off another piece, penetrating my A-3 jacket, heated suit, shirt, underwear, and then opened my skin. I was lucky that it didn't hit any of the electric wires in my suit.

To sum it up you can say — flak suit saves gunner from serious injury. Fellows — wear that flak suit. I can't write anything that may impress you more, so I'll say again "Flak suit, I love you."[6]

Morale fluctuated significantly with each casualty. As a general rule, mental-health issues stemmed less from the prospect of killing the enemy and more from concern about surviving missions and the fear of losing a life within the squadron. Bad weather caused inactivity, which also negatively affected the mental health of the men. When the English weather was bad, as it was in March 1944, it prevented aerial practice and the crews became restless. That restlessness compounded by the gloom of heavy clouds, mist, rain, and constant wind led to feelings of depression.

At one point during the war, each man was allowed to return stateside after flying a minimum of fifty missions. Eventually, however, this mandate was cancelled due to a shortage of experienced men. This change further damaged morale. Numerous crewmen became "flak happy" and only continued into combat through tremendous personal efforts. For some, it was all they could do to have enough courage to leave on another mission. After they had flown thirty missions, the problem of fatigue affected 60 to 65 percent of the combat crews. (Indications of occupational fatigue included irritability, sleeplessness, and battle dreams.) Per the new revocation of the fifty-mission policy, Lamb would issue week-long passes to the men between their twenty-fifth and thirtieth missions and two-week-long passes between their fortieth and fiftieth missions. This plan did have a positive effect on morale. If it was necessary for Lamb to send a pilot to a rest home at any time, this policy did not apply.

Medical board interviews were held to determine the sanity of soldiers. The board was composed of three flight surgeons, all captains. One captain was designated president and another as recorder of the board while it convened. These flight surgeons were usually general practitioners; only a few specialized in psychiatry. During one such court-martial case, the board determined that the soldier was sane—in a continual psychopathic sate and a pathological liar, but sane. Lamb was appointed to serve as a member of this board during a special court-martial at Station #492 in April 1944.

When crew members received time off, they generally spent their R&R in a set number of places. One of these was in Torquay, England, where there was a rest and relaxation camp. Located on the southeastern coast of the country, Torquay was known for its healthy air and was dubbed the "English Riviera."

Another popular location was Hillersbauch Rest Center in southern England. A pleasure-filled place, it had been a resort hotel before the war but had since been taken over as an R&R spot. There the men could enjoy a pool, tennis courts, horseback riding with laid-out bridle paths, movies, hot showers, real food—no K rations—a laundry, cold beer, coke, paper for writing letters, and medical care.

Lamb attended regular continuing-education seminars on medical topics while stationed in England. He was sent by special order written March 17, 1944, to a meeting of the American Medical Society at the Eastern Base Section. Topics for discussion during these gatherings included subjects like lower back pain, fractures of the femur, knee-joint derangement, dyspepsia, and the latest use of penicillin. There were also conversations about psychotic issues, combat exhaustion, and chemical warfare. Lamb appreciated these meetings and took pleasure in attending. As he wrote in a letter home, "I recently went to a medical meeting at one of the General hospitals and enjoyed the lectures very much."

When a flight surgeon left to attend meetings like these—or to go to a school, such as the Eighth Air Force Provisional Medical Field Service School at Station #101— another flight surgeon would be appointed as acting group surgeon during his absence. These school sessions could last as long as two weeks. Lamb listened attentively to the lectures offered while he attended these meetings, but more importantly he passed information on to crew members through his own talks once he returned to the squadron. It took continuous learning, sharing of his knowledge, and all of Lamb's skill as a doctor to help keep the pilots well and the planes in the air as the IX Troop Carrier Command prepared for the invasion of Normandy.

Chapter Seven
Preparing to Invade

The pilots of the IX Troop Carrier Command and the paratroopers of the 101st Airborne had no idea when or where the Normandy invasion would occur, but their days during the winter and early spring of 1944 were spent practicing and preparing for the offensive. From January to May, their emphasis was placed on making two-hour to two-and-a-half-hour flights, which was the time it would take to fly to the Normandy coast. Meanwhile, the glider pilots concentrated on flying and landing heavily loaded gliders.

The lessons learned during the invasion of Sicily and later Italy produced important changes: 1) Operational planners became permanent staff; 2) Coordination between airborne and troop carrier commands became a priority; 3) The pilots would be rigorously trained to fly at night, in bad weather, and in close formation; and 4) Pathfinders would be organized to go ahead of troop carriers and mark drop zones. Pathfinders were a new concept at this point in the war. A handful of specially trained paratroopers, they dropped behind enemy lines earlier than other paratroopers in order to set up drop zones for the larger group. To ensure that the troops landed in a concentrated pattern in the correct location, Pathfinders marked parachute and glider drop zones using visual and navigational aids.

The pilots repeatedly flew in low-level formations with gliders in tow. Along with the beautiful spring-green countryside of England came bad weather. It was often foul, with wind gusts up to twenty miles per hour. This "socked in" the fields, but pilots flew whenever the skies cleared. As the weather permitted or the fog lifted, full training operations were carried out, including towing Waco CG-4A and Airspeed Horsa gliders in both day and night formations while making constant modifications to the C-47s. Practice missions were coordinated with the airborne and gliderborne troopers in as many different weather conditions as possible to simulate actual expected situations.

Ground crews and air crews worked around the clock to keep planes in top condition. Usually only 140-50 C-47s of a wing of just less than 200 were operational at any given time. Gliders were moved by jeeps to the runway. Each tow rope had to be inspected, with special attention given to the rings at the ends used to attach the glider to the plane.

A pilot's day consisted of flying, preparing for his next flight, and attending briefings with the glider troopers before fights. By the end of a day, pilots were exhausted.

Lamb was still in Sicily when a detailed order was issued stating what was expected of the IX Troop Carrier Command's involvement with the invasion of Normandy. The order specified the major activity in IX TCC was to relate to training. A field order of November 9, 1943, ordered the 50th Troop Carrier Squadron (TCS) to undertake full-scale training missions, and on November 18 troop carriers and gliders of the 52nd wing carried 395 British paratroopers in a rehearsal of cross-channel operations. In December, the operation known as "regimental combat team exercises" began. These were elaborately planned training exercises involving as many battle techniques of air transportation as possible, including nightly re-supply missions and operations employing combined paratroopers and gliders for each tow aircraft.

New men were joining the IX TCC regularly, and crew integrity was affected by each new plane and new man. New members did not share the history of the rest of the group, making integrating them difficult. By May, there were twice as many planes available as there had been when the IX TCC was in Africa, and training escalated to a maddening pace. They grew to fourteen troop carrier groups, becoming six times larger than they had been in Africa.

Every member of the command felt the pain of long days and long hours, from the pilots and mechanics all the way down to the men supplying the food. The swelling number of troops, which would increase to over a million by the end of May, made living conditions difficult. Mess hall lines were long because the food-service men were not prepared for the rapid influx of new troops. Except at mess halls in the field (where troops used their mess kits when they ate), porcelain or china plates were usually used at mealtime; these plates required hand-washing by the kitchen staff and took time to replenish. The larger the number of men in the camp, the longer it took to prepare these dishes and the longer the men would have to wait to eat. The increase in the number of men also made Lamb's job more difficult; he was required to be available twenty-four hours a day.

As the staging area for the invasion, southern England

became a gigantic armed camp. Airdromes were plentiful and the sky busy. Runways seemed to be everywhere and pilots had to be careful. All units were regularly resupplied with C-47- and C-53-type transport and cargo planes.

Army personnel were housed everywhere. Trucks, tanks, jeeps, and additional Army vehicles were parked in the forests. Various aircraft, including gliders, covered all flat strips of land and every corner of the airfield. Long convoys of trucks and rail trains carried supplies to the coast day and night. Ships of all types and sizes packed the Port of Southampton, all in preparation for the invasion.

By April 1944, the Allies had broken the back of the German Luftwaffe and were heavily bombing marshalling yards as a first priority. The secondary targets were pilotless bombs, or V-1s, and then airfields. Enemy batteries were located and designated as targets along the coast of northern France. These were bombed from Dunkirk in the Pas-de-Calais area to the Carentan Peninsula to the south. Germany provided regular radio propaganda to the Allied camps in England; the Germans seemed to fear Patton.

That same month, all aircrews were required to have photographs taken of themselves wearing civilian clothes. These pictures would be used for escape purposes, if necessary. The squadrons also set up a defense platoon to guard the base.

On April 8, the pilots of the 50th TCS dropped sixty-three British troopers in Operation Dorothy, simulating the invasion. April 9 and 10 were spent in formation-flying and glider-towing practice. Full night missions were flown, setting up formations and landing gliders in a mass of other planes. These missions included drops of both British and American paratroopers. On April 21-23, the IX TCC rehearsed an English Channel crossing. They made use of their training when fifty-four aircraft were used to drop British troopers in Operation Mush. The flight lasted two hours and ten minutes, the exact length of time it took to fly from Membury, England, to Normandy. The large, loud, and powerful planes pulling gliders came close to the ground, just over the tree tops. This agitated the livestock in the area. Animals were known to run into each other and into buildings; during one exercise a plane flew so low that a nurse on the beach was decapitated by a propeller.

There were a number of other accidents during those training months. One night, a British paratrooper became tangled in the shroud lines as he went out the door of the plane. No rescue was possible. He was cut loose over the "wash" [water] and later picked up by the air-sea rescue. During one night mission, two planes collided in mid-air. Twelve men lost their lives, including a commanding officer and a chaplain. In late spring, a group of fifteen men who had recently trained as Pathfinders crashed. These men were specifically schooled in setting up signals that alerted pilots to supply drop areas. The loss of them and their skills was keenly felt. One of the most unfortunate and senseless accidents occurred when two pilots of a group became drunk and got into a fight. Their disagreement carried over into the next day while they were each piloting their own planes in the same formation. One pilot touched the other's wing, the second pilot touched back, and both planes crashed, killing twelve men.

As the troops continued to train through mid-April, their senses were heightened that the invasion was not far off. At one point they were restricted to camp, which increased speculation that it might be time, but the restriction was lifted five day later.

Diplomats faced travel restrictions as England began preparations for invasion. The British War Cabinet clamped down on diplomatic privileges, held up diplomatic bags, and put all foreign embassies under surveillance.

On April 26, 1944, the publication of the "Ninth Air Force Tactical Air Plan for operation Neptune" was released. It contained 1,300 legal-size pages, including 100 maps and charts. The invading assembly was the largest tactical air force ever to work as a unit. This tactical plan was modified many times before the "go" order was given. On that same day, part of the group flew or towed new gliders from Aldermoston and Greenham Common, adding to the mass of planes already stationed at the field. During the last week in April, more than six hundred American soldiers and sailors died during a training exercise code-named Tiger after being attacked by German motor torpedo boats in the English Channel.

May 1944's flight schedule was hectic. On May 5, IX TCC Headquarters initiated a different kind of exercise. It was announced that only combat crews were permitted forty-eight hour passes; those passes were issued, but they were canceled shortly thereafter. This was Headquarters' way of simulating what would be necessary to get crews back to the fields and to judge the time required to do so.

All-out aerial assaults began on enemy communications

in any country in Europe that Germany held. Train stations, road and rail bridges, radar installations, wireless telegraph stations, and power transformations within a 150-mile radius of the Normandy coastline were targeted.

Lamb knew the invasion was drawing near but not where the troops would land. By late May, troopers were put behind fenced-in areas and guarded. They received plenty of good food and rest. During the weeks leading up to D-Day, which was the day that the force would invade France, Lamb continued his regular duties, making sure the men were healthy enough for the mission. Some pilots had to be grounded because they had respiratory infections. Shortly before D-Day, all medical officers were certified in the use of .45 caliber pistols and carbines. Despite Geneva Convention stipulations that medical personnel should not carry firearms, Lamb was ordered to have a pistol with him on D-Day.

The initial briefing of upper-level officers took place on May 31. Maj. Gen. Paul L. Williams, commanding officer of the IX Troop Carrier Command, found the 50th TCS trained and ready to go for D-Day. Many of the men were veterans of the invasion in the Mediterranean. Williams stated that Maj. Joseph McClure had worked the 50th into an organized, efficient unit despite the English weather.

During the first few days of June 1944, the base was sealed. Station defense was out in force, but minor breaches still occurred. All travel was banned. Men were restricted to base both day and night for a week with no visitors allowed. No outgoing phone calls were permitted. Incoming and outgoing personal mail was stored. There was a guard posted at the squadron room and group intelligence room doors. The secret was out—it was "go" time.

Combat crews were sequestered from the rest of the squadron. Non-combat troops (including officers) were moved out of crew barracks to barracks surrounded by barbed wire and put under twenty-four-hour guard. The combat crews all ate in the Officers' Mess. Breakfast included real eggs, bacon, toast, and coffee. Lunch featured roasted chicken. Steak was the main dish for supper. Pilots made a point of eating a large meal before going on a mission because they never knew when their next meal would be available.

On June 3, men were restricted to station at 0500, as were the crew chiefs, radio operators, and navigators. There was one navigator per three planes. After the preliminary briefing that morning, the word started to leak out—the invasion was on.

A pilot remarked after this meeting that the flight surgeon had "hovered" over the aircrews like a mother hen, ascertaining if their physical and mental conditions would allow them to fly.

On June 4, the invasion was cancelled for twenty-four hours due to inclement weather. Thirty minutes before the pilots' briefing for Operation Neptune-Bigot, the 50th TCS's invasion code name, the mission was postponed. Pilots were under heavy stress and felt the nerve-wracking pressure to ensure that nothing went wrong. They could not afford a disaster. Tensions ran high, as the delay meant the Germans would have time to further fortify the coastline.

General Eisenhower had decided, based on moonlight

and tide reports, that June 5 was the best day to invade. Instead, that day was spent by Intelligence and Operations Sections getting and giving all information possible to crew members. Maps, escape kits, purses, and overlays were issued and planes readied. While it was still raining, maintenance was ordered to paint three white stripes, each two feet wide, on the topside and the underside of the wings of each plane and glider just outside and parallel with the plane's cabin. Brooms and mops were used when the paint brushes gave out. The same three stripes were painted around the aircraft just forward of the tail section, creating zebra striping, or invasion stripes. These were the identifying markers to help invasion forces quickly recognize whether

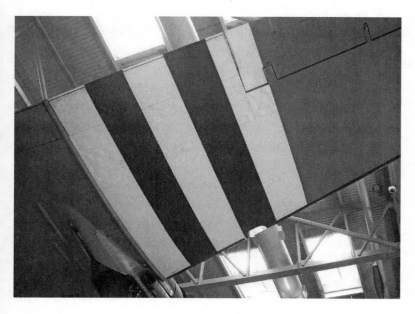

Invasion stripes on a C-47

or not an aircraft was friend or enemy. Aircraft without white stripes would be shot out of the air with no questions asked. The stripes were used to identify Allied planes in an effort to prevent the same friendly fire that had downed so many troop carrier aircraft during the Sicily invasion.

With no need for further delay, the mission proceeded on June 6, 1944. The events of the day began early, as noted by flight surgeon Samuel T Moore:

> Today is D-DAY!!!!! This is the day we have all been waiting for. We were gotten out of the sack at 00.30 hrs. this Tuesday, and alerted for enemy action. Everyone on the base was under arms, tense and excited. The station defense was out in force and most of us were more afraid of trigger happy defense boys than we were of enemy action. [Weather] briefing was at 01.00 hrs. for pilots only and the target was secret.[1]

After this early-morning weather briefing, paratroopers were separated from the other men in the camp. In ignorance of what was to come, the average paratrooper prepared his gear as he had been trained. The rest of the camp buzzed with activity as preparations were made for the invasion. Equipment was checked and re-checked by the flight crew and the maintenance crews, the planes were inspected, and the flight plans reviewed again and again. Pilots took time to eat well and rest, as it would be hours before they had another good meal or the opportunity to take it easy.

Finally, at 2000 hours, crews due to participate in Operation Neptune-Bigot were briefed and missing overlays were prepared. Security and secrecy remained essential. Guards surrounded the briefing rooms and credentials had to be shown to enter. Only pilots were briefed, but the drop area was kept secret even from them until two hours before takeoff. The crews went directly to their planes after the briefing, at about 2200 hours. They had to wait by the planes until it was time to board. Crews were not told their destination until the engines of the planes were started. After long months of preparation, the 314th Troop Carrier Group's two hundred C-47s waited in closely packed lines on the runway. Except for the sounds of the plane engines warming up, there was little noise that summer morning.

Some of the men were superstitious about their planes and who flew with them. Buck Buchanan, one such pilot in the 50th TCS and a friend of Lamb's, foresaw tragedy when he learned that one of his comrades would be flying with him. "I also had a premonition when Sid Dunagan boarded the truck taking us to our ships on our first trip over Normandy," he wrote. Unfortunately, Buchanan's

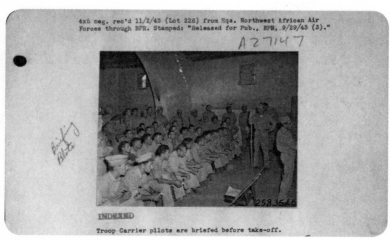

Briefing pilots for the mission

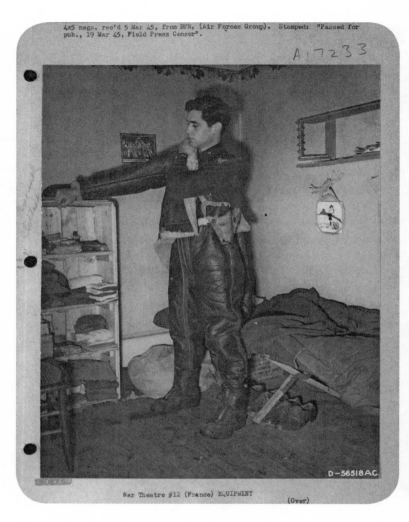

Pilot getting dressed in preparation for the invasion

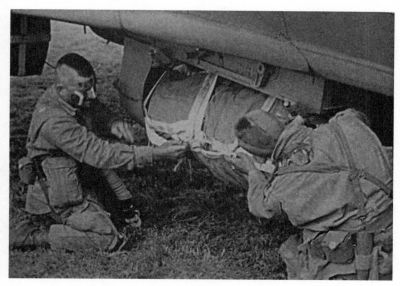

Parapacks being loaded into a C-47

foreboding sense was warranted, as "Sid was the only fatality on that flight."[2]

A pilot in the 81st Troop Carrier Squadron prepared carefully for take off, documented step-by-step:

> The pilot looked at the status card, walked around the AT-6 looking at hinges on the ailerons, elevators, and the rudder. He opened the petcock under the gas tanks, drained out a little liquid on his fingers and smelled his hands. "Good man, Sarge. No water in there. I sure as hell don't need a slug of water in the engine about the time I'm halfway thru a slow roll. . . ." The Lieutenant crawled into the front cockpit and I in the back. The pilot adjusted his safety belt, uncaged the instruments and started the engine. A ground crew member pulled away the wheel chocks. As the pilot taxied out toward the active runway his friend followed in another AT-6.

At the end of Runway 19 the pilot turned facing at a forty-five degree angle toward incoming traffic, set the brakes and opened up the throttle. The engine roared and settled down into a steady throb of power while the aircraft strained against the brakes. He pushed the propeller pitch control to low pitch/high rpm and repeated the cycle to be sure the pitch control was working. He switched off one magneto and carefully noted the slight rpm drop. He moved all the controls through full deflection to be sure they were free and smooth.

The pilot snugged up his safety belt, switched the radio to the Maxwell control tower frequency and called the tower.

"AT Six zero-two-six-five-niner ready for take-off on one-niner, over."

The tower controller replies, "AT Six five niner, what is your intention, over?"

"Tower AT Six, five-niner and AT Six seven-one-three-five-niner request permission to take off on runway one-niner for a workout in the local area."

"Make a turn to the right to a heading of two-seven-zero degrees for your climb out as soon as practical after clearing the boundaries, over."

"Roger, tower. Understand take off on one-niner, turn to two-seven-zero for climb out. Wilco, out."[3]

The pilots of the 50th TCS taxied their C-47s out onto the six-thousand-foot runway and opened up the throttle as they turned. When the order came at about 2230 hours, troop carrier planes began their takeoffs in radio silence. The first plane rolled down the runway, picking up speed. As it approached takeoff speed, the pilot gently pulled back on the stick and maintained the directional control with the rudders. The plane lifted off. Dust, weeds, and grass whipped up by propellers flew up and back over the gliders. The C-47 settled and then started a steady climb.

The 314th and 315th Troop Carrier Groups based in Grantham took off in nearly zero visibility and flew through a cloud deck to approximately nine thousand feet. The first plane in line had the shortest runway and the most difficult time getting into the air. That pilot had to "sweat it out" until he pulled up and lifted off. Planes took off according to a precise timetable, and each air station was assigned a degree of ascent so there would be no collisions. There was a twenty-second interval between takeoffs as the C-47s formed standard V formations in groups of nine. The formations of nine circled in a holding pattern until the last of the nearly two hundred planes was in the air, by which time the lead C-47 was miles away. The whole process took

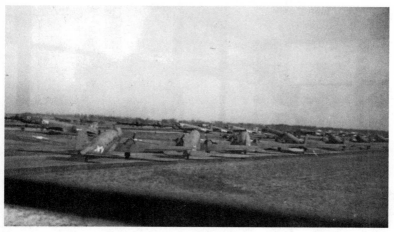

Planes prepared to take off for the invasion

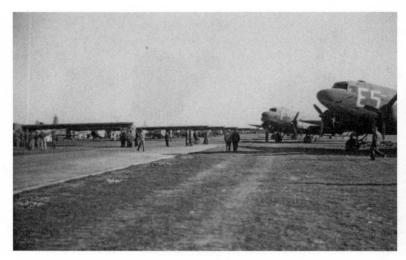

Planes prepared to take off for the invasion

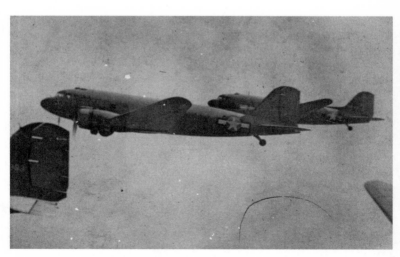

C-47s flying in formation

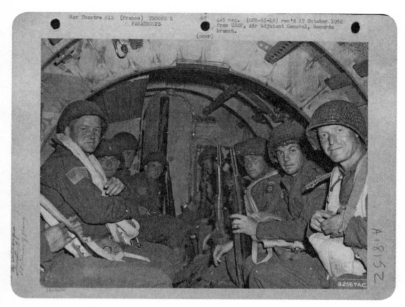

Paratroopers prepared to jump from a C-47

an hour and a half to execute. The American-piloted planes continued circling until they formed an 850-plane formation that included the eighteen planes of the 50th Squadron.

From thousands of feet below, all Lamb could see in the night sky were plane lights. The glow of the planes in V formations reminded him of a Christmas tree. It was an awesome sight. Aircraft filled the sky. Right and left, front and back, there were thousands—a skytrain miles long.

Per orders from his superiors, Lamb had become invested in the lives of the crews in those planes. After living with them day in and day out, he got to know them on a personal level and had formed an emotional bond with each man. With a heavy heart and a mountain of hope, Lamb began the long, agonizing wait for the planes to return.

Chapter Eight
D-Day

As a whole, the Normandy invasion operation, enormous in scale, was code-named Operation Overlord. Operation Torch, the invasion of Sicily in which the IX TCC participated, had involved a battalion-size airborne assault. The Normandy invasion was much larger in scale. The Allied force leaving Britain comprised six seaborne divisions — three US, two British, and one Canadian — that landed on five beachheads. In addition, there were three airborne divisions, two US and one British.

The D-Day force included 14,130 aircraft: 1,030 gliders, 1,700 medium and light bombers, 3,500 heavy bombers, 5,500 fighter planes, and 2,400 C-47 transport planes. The Allies had 160,000 men in three airborne and six infantry divisions that included armored and commando units. The Navy's fleet of nearly 5,300 vessels consisted of 5 battle ships, 23 cruisers, 2,700 troopships, and 2,500 landing craft. Their contribution to the invasion force also included 150,000 men and 1,500 tanks.

Operation Bigot was the code name for the air portion of the invasion force. The landing invasion on the northern coast of Normandy, east of Cherbourg, was given the code name Operation Neptune.

German Gen. Erwin Rommel had overseen the heavy

fortification of the coast of France and the surrounding area. Rommel's defenses were referred to as Hitler's "Atlantic Wall." Hitler believed the invasion would occur near Pas-de-Calais, on the northern part of the coastline. This was a critical error that caused German forces to be taken completely by surprise. In addition, bad weather in the first few days of June made the German Navy cancel its normal patrols of the English Channel.

The Allies had bombed the German batteries located along the coast of northern France in preparation for D-Day, but there were still five German panzer divisions and thirty-two infantry divisions waiting. They were scattered between Rotterdam, in the Netherlands, and the peninsula of France. The Allies were putting thirty-seven divisions up against sixty divisions the Germans had stationed on the western front.

All fourteen groups of the IX Troop Carrier Command took part in the opening move of the offensive. As recorded in the 50th Troop Carrier Squadron's monthly report for May 1944, this included the participation of 49 officers, 239 enlisted men, and 21 airplanes of the 50th TCS. The squadron's job was to deliver parachute- and glider-borne infantry of the 82nd and 101st Airborne Divisions to six drop zones (or landing zones) in close proximity to Sainte-Mère-Église from midnight to the early morning.

The paratroopers' mission was to arrive hours before the seaborne invasion to seize bridges, roads, and other key points. They were also to assist the inland progress of the assault troops landing on Utah Beach and to prevent a German counterattack.

Lamb stood with his heart in his throat as the IX TCC

thundered off into the night and headed east to the continent. In the official 314th Troop Carrier Group report it was written that between 2338 hours on June 5, 1944, and 0540 hours on June 6, 1944, Quinn Corley lead eighteen C-47s of the 50th TCS carrying paratroopers from Saltby. These C-47s would join planes that took off from Melbury and four other fields, assembling forty miles south of Reading. The 50th Troop Carrier Squadron had a three-part mission on D-Day: 1) Deliver paratroopers; 2) Deliver gliders full of troops; 3) Deliver supplies.

The weather was overcast up to 5,000 feet at liftoff. Near the English Channel, C-47s and gliders from other fields joined the glider stream. On a 195-degree heading, the planes descended to 1,000 feet and stayed steady for twenty-nine miles, over water.

Four minutes after the planes passed checkpoint Flatbush along the English coast, the navigation lights and amber recognition lights still remained on. The pilots maintained this heading for fifty-seven more miles to a point code-named Hoboken, which was a ship in the English Channel west of the Bailiwick of Guernsey. There the planes changed their course and moved toward the coast of the Cherbourg Peninsula. At that point, the amber lights were extinguished and the blue formation lights were turned to the lowest practical intensity. Even exhaust flames were dampened; this was achieved by slipping a manufactured pipe over the exhaust, which the crew did before they left the airfield. The final, fifteen-minute leg of the crossing began. As they neared land, the planes descended to an altitude of 700 feet in order to stay below German radar.

Navigation for this invasion was easier for the pilots

in Lamb's group than what they had experienced when flying to Sicily. This time the flight route was planned, so the pilots received radio and light signals every thirty miles. Even boats in the English Channel were fitted with lights marking the pilots' direction. Below the swarm of planes was the naval invasion force of battleships, cruisers, destroyers, and troopships—all moving in unison toward the French coast.

In an account given by one pilot, the rain had stopped and the moon was shining by the time his plane reached the Normandy coast. As the sky cleared, the planes flew south. The paratroopers had been loud and aggressive as they loaded the plane with their heavy packs and other supplies. Their energy continued during the flight, but they were sobered as the drop zone approached. There had been no enemy opposition until the plane reached the west coast of the Cherbourg Peninsula. Luckily it flew through with no damage and arrived at the drop zone.

Still, while in flight the planes flew into cloudbanks, which required them to use instrument-only navigation. It was even noted in the 50th War Diary that Maj. Joseph H. McClure (RAF Saltby), who was attached to the 50th TCS, hit clouds and flew in zero visibility. Without radio contact, he wandered off, but he returned without incident. One glider pilot noted that his aircraft passed through the clouds at 120 miles per hour. He felt a little buffeting but nothing truly alarming. He had wished that the C-47 pilot would slow down a little nonetheless, but he had no way to communicate with the tow plane.

One view of operations came from Col. Charles H. Young,

commander of the 439th TCG, who led the 50th Troop
Carrier Wing by flying his radar C-47:

> The 439th had arrived at stations at 2200 hours, take offs
> had started at 2313, and the regular troop carrier route to
> Normandy was followed. The horseman guiding his steed
> sideways to get him squared away for his jump over a high
> bar and broad pit, the turning, loosens the reins and feels the
> surge of power ripple through his spirited mount, knows
> something of how I felt on the night of June 5th/6th as I
> turned out of the formation of 81 troop carrier C-47s at the
> last check point in the English Channel, leading in the first
> group of the 50th Troop Carrier Wing, and started on the
> final straight run-in to the German held Normandy. Not that
> I'm kidding myself about the lumbering old C-47 Skytrains
> being powerful or spirited, but the potent fighting cargo we
> carried, the eager tough young paratroopers of Colonel Sink
> of the 101st Airborne Division, gave us that sense of power
> and spirit.[1]

One by one, the C-47s arrived at Normandy, pilots and
paratroopers alike acutely conscious of their mission. Many
took enemy fire before they reached France, some reporting
tracers from batteries on the Channel Islands. Heavy,
intense, accurate fire was also reported for a full mile east
of Sainte-Mère-Église. One crew member marveled at the
way any of the planes headed for Normandy were able
to reach their drop zones successfully. The bright red and
green lights from the tracers came at the planes through
the ground-based searchlight beams; there were so many
tracers and so many planes, he did not understand how
even one of the aircraft was missed. Despite the ack-ack,
another term for flak, the pilots held the plane straight and
steady, allowing the paratroopers to jump.

Hostile fire inspired varied reactions in the crewmen. "While going into the DZ [drop zone], some displayed extreme excitement," remembered Col. Joseph Harkiewicz of the 29th TCS. At the same time, "the veteran pilots quickly drew their attention from the enemy fire and into the cockpit, soothing the atmosphere with calm instructions.[2] One crew member of the 50th TCS had this to say about the troops in his plane that morning: "Paratroopers found their voices, with first warning of drop zone ahead, ready to jump, they worked themselves up into bedlam pitch. Some were quiet as they jumped, others bellowed and others wise-cracked. Germans were shooting in earnest. The end of the line was not as eager to go, some had to be 'helped.'"[3] In his book *Brave Men*, Ernie Pyle describes his own fear as he prepared to face the force awaiting the Allies on the beaches of Normandy: "From a vague anticipatory dread the invasion now turned into a horrible reality to me. In a matter of hours the holocaust of our own planning would swirl over us. No man could guarantee his own fate."[4]

Three planes in one troop carrier squadron fell to enemy fire, but only after dropping their paratroopers. Of course, not all planes involved in the mission were as successful. A pilot reported seeing a plane go down in flames; the plane was lost, along with the crew and eighteen British paratroopers. Another account told of a plane returning from the Cherbourg Peninsula on one engine, having limped back after throwing overboard anything that was not tied down. Those who returned safely were humbled by the experience. "The fire on our right and left looked like so many lighted tennis balls; however their beauty did not blot out the death message they carried. If you saw one standing still, it had your number," recalled a pilot of the 50th TCS. "Off, full bore, like a scalded dog, planes were going down around us and I was sure we would be next. The gray dawn was peeping over the horizon. When we reached Folkingham we both agreed there was no future in flying."[5]

Flying over German-controlled land was one of the most dangerous and physically demanding tasks of the entire war. All air group personnel were considered nonexpendable. They had to live to fight again, and airplanes were not easily replaced. Significant money and time had gone into building the planes and training the crews.

The TCC utilized a delivery formation of nine aircraft known as the "V of Vs." Visually similar to a flock of geese flying, this formation divided the nine planes into three clusters of three, each three-plane group arranged in a V shape. Together, the three clusters flew in a larger V shape relative to one another. The V of Vs was designed to put the aircraft in the closest proximity to each other and avoid turbulence from preceding aircraft. This type of flight, in which paratroopers were delivered to jump zones, was called a serial; the only way to drop paratroopers close together is for the aircraft to fly close together and release them at nearly the same time, which is why the V of V formation was selected.

When the pilots found themselves in the clouds on D-Day, the integrity of much of their formations was lost. Because of this, many groups of paratroopers were scattered around the Cherbourg Peninsula. Some paratroopers missed their drop zones by as much as twenty miles. This was not from lack of training in night formation or combat experience. There are many stories of flight crews turning around and making return passes over their drop zones to drop their troops while under enemy fire.

After fifteen months of glider-towing training, the C-47 pilots joined their formation with confidence and skill. The planes sometimes pulled gliders in tandem. These pilots were responsible for their plane and crew along with the gliders they towed filled with paratroopers, as well as navigation and communication equipment. American airmen felt superior to the enemy and believed they were doing something great. They had trained and knew their jobs well. "The mighty host was tense as a coiled spring," a pilot recalled, quoting General Eisenhower. After days and weeks of working toward this point, the pilots were both anxious and relieved to be finally flying this mission.

The 50th TCS's mission of delivering the 82nd Airborne had a sub-code name of Boston, a component of the larger-scale Operation Neptune. The first paratroopers were dropped at 0015 hours. A full "stick" of twenty-eight paratroopers from the Regimental Headquarters Company, the 508th Parachute Infantry, and Task Force A of the 82nd Airborne Division was one of the groups dropped over France by a C-47 of the 50th TCS. Two hours after leaving England, 13,000 paratroopers had parachuted out of planes over France. Gliders with full, heavy loads had also been released from the C-47s. Glider pilots chose the best spots to land their loads of men, jeeps, mortars, and shells. One hundred gliders found their predetermined landing zones.

A Horsa glider could carry a load of up to 7,200 pounds of artillery and ammunition, plus the pilot and co-pilot. The glider itself could physically carry even more weight than this, but it was already a heavy load for a C-47. Other gliders might carry a jeep and two men, a 75mm pack howitzer, or a full load of glider-borne troops with full packs. Troops in full battle gear, which weighed almost as much as they did, could weigh in at 340-60 pounds per person.

During that first morning, the 50th TCS delivered 319 paratroopers, 1,868 pounds of ammunition, and thousands of pounds of combat equipment. Eighty percent of the troops and supply bundles landed within a mile of the drop zones. The 50th War Diary documents the squadron's success in their mission. It is noted: "Returned at 0540, 6 June. All aircraft returned." They had helped spearhead the invasion and had done their job well. Adrenaline rushing, the pilots returned excited about the mission and boisterously congratulating each other. Intelligence officers, intent on gathering as much information about the mission as possible, wanted to know exactly where each of the planes had dropped men, where the flak positions were located, and where distressed aircraft were sighted.

The types of medical injuries reported after the invasion included a broken left arm, an eye injury, and leg injuries. One crew member had broken both legs. A pilot from the 50th TCS was taken to the general hospital five miles from the base at 1630 for attention to a minor wound. Curious how the pilot had come by his injuries, the emergency doctor asked, "What've you been doing?" "Dropping paratroopers, Sir," the pilot answered. "The invasion is on." The doctor looked at him in disbelief; he had no idea. The Normandy invasion was not officially announced until 1830.

At headquarters, Lamb received a radio message that a pilot of a plane had been killed. The first lieutenant had been shot in the left side of his chest with a small caliber gun. This lieutenant had turned around and made a second pass over the drop zone, putting out two paratroopers who had become tangled and couldn't make it out during the first pass. By the time the lieutenant had turned the large plane, German gunfire had become heavy. Internal bleeding resulted in the pilot's death a few minutes later as he was coming off the drop zone after a second pass.

During those early days of the invasion, caring for the wounded was a matter of being creative. Operating tables or beds were often stretchers set on two sawhorses of equal height. Seeing that the bandages of the wounded were changed was a regular detail Lamb was responsible for. He checked each man as he returned for any unusual reaction to the mission. He administered a double shot of rye to take the edge off the hyper pilots and crews. The usual coffee and sandwiches were waiting as well. Not surprisingly, many of the men of the 50th TCS exhibited signs of stress upon their return. Lamb looked for the usual, visible signs of stress, mainly trembling hands, shaking, and insomnia. The wind was raw during the flight—too cold for a man to sweat, yet many did. Delayed reactions were normal, and some men who had held themselves together throughout the course of the mission began to crumble once they returned to safety. Men were worried about those who had not returned, their anxiety for missing comrades manifesting itself physically.

To add to the tension, men reported missing would sometimes turn up days later, maybe washing up on the beach dead. Of course, there was also concern among the pilots of the 50th TCS about what was happening back in France when they were not flying.

The apprehension and general uneasiness of Lamb's men upon returning to base were shared by crewmen of other troop carrier squadrons. "Once you get over it and are on the ground you start thinking about the others," acknowledged one man from the 81st TCS. "I don't know what happened. When I got back to the barracks I couldn't keep my legs still, no matter what. . . . Did I do alright? Then proud that I was part of the big invasion. . . . How many saw me shake? What will they think of me in the morning?"[6]

Once the pilots had the planes on the ground again, they, along with their crews, made a cursory examination of the aircraft, looking for any battle damage. All were surprised that only half of the aircraft had been hit. Damage ranged from harmless bullet holes to heavy structural losses that could have caused the planes to crash in flames at the drop zone. Six planes were damaged enough to be non-flyable. All pilots stated they dropped at their designated drop zone or vicinity.

After the debriefing, the cook served the crew fresh eggs, bacon, pancakes, French toast, and pineapple juice, which was a special treat. Pineapple juice was hard to come by, and the sugar in it served as a welcome pick-me-up for the men. Empty seats in the dining room were a sinister reminder of losses after a mission. Exhausted, the flight crews went to bed while the mechanics and their crews feverishly worked on the damaged aircraft to prepare them for the next mission.

Now the isolated airborne units had to be resupplied. The priority items had to go by air; that would be the 314th's next mission. At 1530 on D-Day—a few hours after the first mission—the aircraft crews of the 50th TCS were assembled for a briefing about resupplying the ground troops. Eighteen planes left at 0330 on the resupply mission, code-named Operation Freeport, and dropped bundles on the Cherbourg Peninsula. The planes of the 50th TCS left on a second resupply trip at 1036 on June 7, or D+1 (the day after the invasion), and returned at 1530. Believing that the worst was over, many men were more confident in this mission than they were the day before. Nonetheless, Operation Freeport presented its own challenges, and once again the squadron suffered losses. One plane crashed, leaving five men missing. An additional three planes did not return, though none were known to have crashed. Eight planes returned damaged.

Despite continued bad weather, a second resupply delivered medical supplies, food, and ammunition to the drop zones. The C-47s that made these trips were provided escort by P-38s and P-47s. On D+2, two days after D-Day, "door bundles" of blood plasma and supplies were pushed out of open cabin doors to supply the 101st Airborne hospital.

The 50th TCS dropped many different kinds of military supplies. The aircraft delivered gasoline, oil, guns, medical equipment, and blankets, anything it took to keep the Army moving. They also continued to pull gliders filled with men and supplies.

At the early-morning start of the invasion on June 6, fully

loaded gliders flew to the front with supplies. Sir Trafford Leigh-Mallory, who commanded the glider force, ruled there would be no glider transport in the daylight because it was too dangerous. Gliders carried airborne officers and large equipment during these missions. Bulldozers were the most dreaded glider load because they were heavy and they often shifted while in flight. In a poor glider landing, a bulldozer could kill more men than German bullets.

Constructed out of canvas and wood, gliders were designed to be disposable and were treated as such. After landing and unloading, the pilots were instructed to work their way to the back line, where they would catch transport to their station to later fly a different glider and perform another mission.

There was a pilot hierarchy within the Army Air Forces. Glider pilots did not receive as much training as other pilots and were required to log forty-two hours as co-pilots in C-47s. The pilots of the C-47s and bombers received the next level of training, while fighter pilots were considered the ultimate flying daredevils.

By mid-June, the 50th squadron was landing on temporary "tarpaper" strips built by airborne engineers with few supplies. Most fields used by the squadron had to be built because there were not enough being liberated to meet the initial demand. Hedgerows and farmland were bulldozed by equipment brought over in gliders. The C-47s arrived to an eternal dust cloud hanging over non-surfaced fields and reloaded to fly out again.

On the return runs, the pilots morphed into "flying ambulance drivers," evacuating hundreds of men to England. Each plane carried twenty-four litters and was similar to an emergency ward. Red Cross markings were used on the return trip when wounded were aboard. Morphine was administered to the patients to help them comfortably make the trip. Often, wounded men arrived with a paper listing their name, rank, serial number, and the field doctor's notes.

The pilots soon had an established routine of supplies in, wounded out. Provisions were flown in, unloaded, the plane refitted for the wounded, and the injured loaded. Normally one doctor and two nurses flew over with the crew. Planes carried both stretcher-bound and ambulatory soldiers.

Robert E. Callahan, a pilot from the 50th TCS, elaborated on the process:

> Not 'till the 11th did we pick up on our supply missions. Now, in most cases, we carried in evac personnel, usually a flight nurse and medical technician. These people were all business. While flying to France, they, like most others in the cabin, napped. While our cargo was being unloaded, the nurse and medic rested away from the activity. However, once the aircraft was unloaded they often pitched in to set up the webbed belts. These hooked from the top of the cabin to the floor, readying them for litters that would be slipped into the openings in the belt, which allowed patients to be stacked four high. The air evac people were tremendous. From the time the ambulances arrived at the aircraft, nurse and medic became different people, all attentive of the physical well-being and spirit of those entrusted to them. They knew just how to talk to the wounded, giving them encouragement without pity. With certainty, many of our troops survived only because of the caring attention of the air evac personnel.[7]

Many crewmen had a difficult time simply observing the wounded; assisting them was an even greater challenge.

Often it caused emotional trauma. Callahan continued with his account of the tragedy pilots on resupply missions witnessed in France:

> A plane load of wounded, in most cases, involved both litter and ambulatory patients. The walking invariably sought out those more serious than they to help. Not at all unusual to see an ambulatory sitting next to a "stump" of a body, the poor soul who lost his arms and legs and was encased in a cast covering his entire body. Holes were made for the eyes and the nose/mouth area. The ambulatory fed beverage to the patient and offered conversation throughout the trip.[8]

From June through September, the 50th squadron flew from Saltby to the continent daily as weather permitted. Lamb continued to work at the hospital in Grantham, focusing on triage and general care of men wounded during the activity in the months following D-Day. On June 26, 1944, he wrote a letter to his family updating them on his post-invasion situation:

> There has been little to write about as far as I am personally concerned. My outfit participated in the earliest stages of the invasion, and our casualties weren't as great as we had anticipated. I was in absolutely no danger myself nor do I expect to be.

> At the present time I am working at a convalescent rest camp for pilots. It is sort of a week's vacation and is rather enjoyable. There is little for me to do. There are horses to ride, swimming, movies, dances, etc. A small dispensary is set up here in the hotel and with another doctor, I only have to work every other day.

> I haven't seen or heard from Betty's brother since the

invasion, but I am anxiously awaiting news from him. I hope to write a more newsy letter if anything ever happens concerning me. I'm idle most of the time as far as medical work is concerned, but hope to get into something soon where there will be more action. Seems that most of the fellows are doing a great deal as compared to me in this mess.

During these first few months, one group of patients Lamb did care for regularly was those who had suffered psychologically after the invasion. He would attend to a planeload of these men per day while they were awaiting air transfer to a hospital in Great Britain. There they would recover enough to be relocated to the States by ship.

Despite the horrors being committed around them, the spirit of most of the aircrews remained rather high. As Ernie Pyle writes in *Brave Men*, these crews had no duties other than flying, and they only flew about two hours a day. Every two weeks, these men received forty-eight hours' leave, which most of them spent in London or nearby cities. "They made friends among the British people, and they looked up those same friends on the next trip to town," explains Pyle. "They did a thousand and one things on their leave, and it did them good. Also, it gradually created an understanding between the two people, a conviction that the other fellow was all right in his own peculiar way."[9]

Not every man handled the stress well, and sometimes these rests were not enough to shield the pilots from mental distress. One account from the Eighth Army Air Force demonstrated how one pilot's workload affected him both emotionally and physically. While a group of pilots were talking, one man, Herb, was asked a question: "When no reply was forthcoming I glanced at Herb and saw that something was seriously wrong. Herb strained to say something but only strangled sound came forth. One side of his face was 'frozen' in place as the other half moved in response to his attempt to speak." The flight surgeon was called in immediately and escorted Herb to the hospital; the doctor determined that "the entire left side of his body was paralyzed as though a switch had been shut off" due to "tension generated by flying gliders in combat." Luckily the damage was not permanent, and Herb was behind the controls in the cockpit again three days later.[10]

After D-Day some of the pilots of the 50th TCS were given leave to go home. Having completed a tour of duty consisting of 750 or more flying hours, these pilots were entitled to a thirty-day pass to the States, excluding travel time, which could be as much as one month to the States and one month back.

The 314th Troop Carrier Group, of which the 50th Troop Carrier Squadron was a part, received the Presidential Unit Citation for the second time for their work during June 5-7, 1944. The citation read: "Accomplished 106 sorties, thereby, distinguishing themselves through extraordinary heroism, determination, and esprit de corps, in a flawlessly coordinated group effort in which troop carrier air planes spearheaded the allied invasion of the European continent."

In July of 1944, missions were flown to France almost daily. Crews were often "stuck" overnight, so they took bed rolls in case they were needed. Supplies delivered by the air crews included camouflage netting, medical supplies, paint, rations, signal corps equipment, coffee, batteries, mortar frames, blood, plasma, gasoline, beans, maps, literature, medals, ammunition, and 5,500 pounds of razor blades (which was only a one-day supply).

Seven hundred tons of gas, rations, and 100mm ammunition were flown to advanced airstrips just behind the front. The amount of freight hauled in August 1944 topped almost 4,000,000 pounds. The same month more than 11,000 battle causalities and 2,500 other patients were flown to medical care.

The 314th TCG also became part of a new command in July called Combined Airborne Forces. Headed by Lt. Gen. Lewis H. Brereton, the command was formed in conjunction with elements of the 82nd Airborne Infantry Division. The 50th TCS took part in a new training program consisting of static loading and unloading, air landing exercises, and two practice paratroop drops.

By this time, pilots were flying to the point of exhaustion. There were three times as many pilots dying from accidents than from enemy action. Untrained and inexperienced medical officers often did not recognize the nature of this type of stress. Lamb's years of experience gave him an advantage over fresher flight surgeons. The medical service's job was to keep the air and ground crews healthy and fit enough to defeat the enemy. It had improved after 1942, and the medical service ultimately succeeded in their assignment. Commanders no longer complained about high rates of sickness that prevented the execution of their assigned missions. Rates of disease and non-battle injuries declined in all theaters. The time Lamb spent in Africa and Sicily helped him excel as a flight surgeon during the months before and after the Normandy invasion. Ninety-seven out of one hundred injured men who made it to an aid station survived. The troops' efficiency was mainly affected by long and hard work hours rather than chronic illness.

On July 26, 1944, almost two months after D-Day, Lamb began to entertain the thought the war may be nearing its end:

> My dearest Mother,
>
> Thanks a lot for your recent letter. Although we haven't been terribly busy lately, I usually find something to do to pass the time away. The countryside is in full bloom nowadays, and it is quite refreshing to cycle out for ten or fifteen miles each afternoon. Especially are the poppy fields in full bloom, and they make quite a pretty site [*sic*].
>
> We have sent many fellows in the outfit home recently and maybe my time will come around someday. Seems that they are still short of doctors over here however, so I'm not expecting it any time soon.
>
> Things are going very well these days and we are beginning to believe now that the war may be over in this area by fall as the Russians seem to really be pouring it on. I have been to [France] and many interesting places lately.
>
> Love to all,

The Allied forces were pushing inland towards Germany, but Lamb's work was not done. It was time to be transferred to a new station in France.

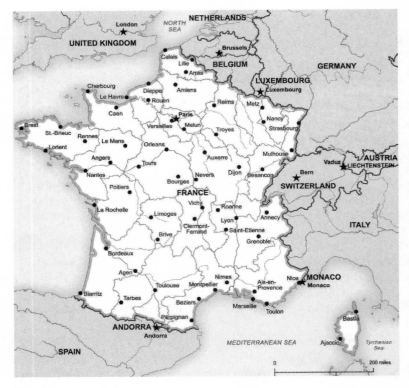

France

Chapter Nine
France

After the initial Normandy invasion on June 6, Allied forces quickly established their operations in France. One of the first necessary steps was to begin constructing airfields and landing strips so pilots could continue delivering supplies and transporting medical personnel. As these fields were named, an "A" before the airfield number indicted that it was an American-engineered field. All airfields build by American engineers had three runways. A "B" was used to designate fields built or made serviceable by the British. Construction on twelve advance airstrips began in June, and seven of these original landing fields became permanently operational. (The other five were abandoned as the troops moved closer to the front, where new airstrips were built as replacements.)

The first field used by the Allies was A-1 at St. Pierre du Mont. The IX TCC landed on this field as they resupplied troops from England. A five-thousand-foot runway right on the beach, it was now used for emergency landings. These landing fields were little more than leveled farm land with a road in the proximity of the strip. The intensive training the IX TCC received in short-field takeoffs and landings during their months in England became invaluable.

These fields were made functional quickly. An engineering

battalion landed on Omaha Beach as early as June 9. They immediately proceeded to the small village of Cardonville. On June 10, the survey party laid out the runway and the tractors began clearing a strip. Grading continued for the next few days. By 6 a.m. on June 14, grading was completed for 50 percent of the runway. The marshaling areas on either end of the runway were also done.

The field in Cardonville was ready for use by June 20. The runway consisted of five thousand feet of heavy wire. This steel-mesh-surfaced runway had two and one half miles of taxi lanes, including truck lanes, and seventy-five hard stands, or areas where the planes were parked just outside of a taxi strip. Amazingly, all of this was accomplished in just ten days with enemy troops nearby.

On June 19, 1944, the IX Troop Carrier Command became the first air force command to operate on the continent. An emergency landing strip was completed at Deux Jumeaux Airfield for immediate use while other fields were being constructed. The 314th TCG moved on to Collerville-sur-Mer and Field A-22, then on to Duex A-3 and A-4 at Poupeville Airfield. Days later, fields were completed at St. Laurent, and by June 25 Carentan A-10 Airfield was being used.

In July 1944, Franklin D. Roosevelt announced that he planned to run for a fourth term as president. That same month, Lamb flew to the 50th TCS field in France. On the envelope of a letter he sent from the camp, he typed the word "France" and then obscured it by typing asterisks over the word. The letters of the word could be seen despite the marks over the country name. This let his mother and family know where he was while circumventing the

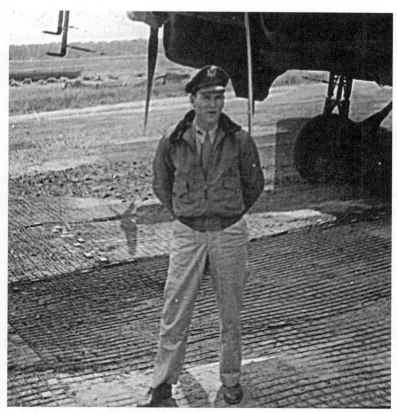

Lamb standing on newly built airfield

censorship officer. He sent the letter airmail through the US Army Postal Service instead of the usual V-mail through the war and Navy departments.

In August 1944, two months after D-Day, Lamb and six aircrews arrived in Poix, France, their new permanent station. Originally an enemy field demolished by the Eighth Air Force earlier in the war, it was used as a base from which the 50th Troop Carrier Squadron supplied the ground troops with food, fuel, and ammunition.

Lamb's first job while stationed at Poix was to see about medical care for men staying in a rest camp. At Poix, he lived in a tent along with his roommate. The advance moving party had already erected tents for Lamb and additional ones for members of the flight crews. The same party established larger tents for operations and units of the squadron, creating a tent city. The two units of the squadron still stationed in England would move to France later in August.

Initially the men were restricted to the base and its immediate vicinity. Later they received passes to the nearby city of Amiens, France, which helped improve morale greatly. Paris surrendered on August 25. With that victory, the men thought the war might be over by the end of the

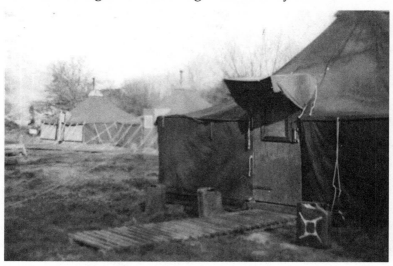

Tents set up in the camp

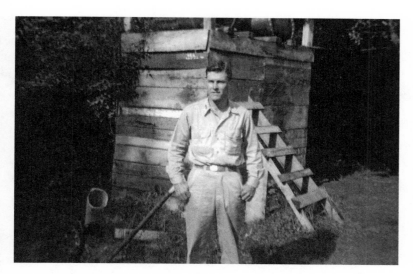

Lamb standing in front of the camp's showers

year. Limited passes began to be issued to Paris. Foster R. Renwick, one of the pilots of the 50th TCS, flew his plane under the Eiffel Tower in his exuberance. Lamb smiled when he shared this bit of information.

One particular type of health issue continued to plague the men—and therefore Lamb as their doctor. In France, VD (particularly gonorrhea) and enlarged prostates were still persistent medical issues. To compound the problem, penicillin was selling on the black market for $200 per vial.

During one medic's check of the first aid boxes in the planes, he discovered that all of the morphine ampoules has been stolen. One of the pilots stated, "It was one of the most disgusting problems our Squadron ever faced." The thief was either addicted to or selling the morphine.

The wet and cold weather also contributed to medical

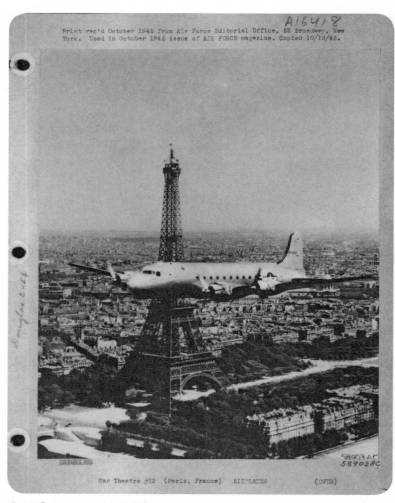

A16418

War Theatre #12 (Paris, France)   AIRPLANES   (OVER)

58903 AC
58903AC

C-47 flying past the Eiffel Tower

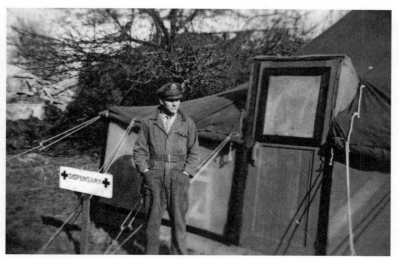

Lamb in front of the camp's dispensary

problems, especially foot issues. A regular diet of C rations added to dysentery concerns. Relapsing fever, food poisoning, beriberi, smallpox, leprosy, ringworm, pneumonia, scabies, lice, hookworms, hepatitis, yaws, dengue fever, bilharzia, and cholera were just a few of the illnesses Lamb treated while he was at Poix.

In France, Lamb faced unusual circumstances that had not been a serious problem in Africa. Here, German soldiers were known to shoot at vehicles and tents with red crosses. It was not unusual for medics to be captured. If possible, Germans would overtake a medical tent and move their ammunition under the cover. The French people, because they lived in a war zone with little food or everyday necessities available, would steal any stores left unattended, including medical supplies.

The men continued to entertain thoughts of the war's end and their return home to America. "Everything these days is encouraging, and it may end in a few weeks," Lamb wrote hopefully on August 26.

> I only hope that plans are made to prevent another war in the future. Surely someone knows the answer.

> Several of our pilots who participated in the recent invasion are now on leave in the states and rumor have it [*sic*] that we may all be home by Xmas. About all anyone thinks about these days is going home. Nothing else seems to matter.

In the fall of 1944, the 50th TCS received their second Air Medal for a job well done during the invasion of Normandy. This time the troops were given oak leaf pins to affix to the ribbon they had already been awarded for their work in Sicily.

There was a general lull in activities that September because fewer supplies were being brought through France. Antwerp, Belgium, had been liberated on September 3. One pilot reported seeing an Allied plane flying between the two steeples of the church in Antwerp in celebration.

German forces still controlled the North Sea around the Port of Antwerp. This created a logistical problem because it necessitated that most of the troop supplies be shipped by air. In order to solve the crisis, General Eisenhower made it a priority to clear the seaward approaches to Antwerp. The plan was to take control of three major waterways in the Netherlands—the Maas, the Waal, and the Lower Rhine—to put the Allies in a position to move through the northern plain of Germany. Code-named Operation Market-Garden, this mission would be the largest air drop in history, with the drop zones as far as eighty-five miles behind enemy lines.

The US 82nd Airborne and 101st Airborne, along with the 1st British and Polish Airborne, were all dropped into Holland, beginning its liberation. The Army's objectives were to control the bridges and roads around the towns of Eindhoven, Nijmegen, and Arnhem and to break through the German defenses in the West. Arnhem, a town on the lower end of the Rhine, was the designated drop zone for the 50th TCS delivering paratroopers.

During daylight hours on September 17, 1944, 72 aircraft of the 314th TCG took off as part of the 550-plane force flying to Arnhem with 1,015 paratroopers and 248 parapack loads of equipment. Each plane could carry six parapacks — collections of supplies that were loaded so that they could be pushed out of the plane and go down by parachute — plus a full load of paratroopers.

In low clouds and heavy fog and under substantial enemy fire, the 50th TCS, led by Lt. Col. Joseph McClure, dropped one of many elements of the 1st British Airborne Division into the vicinity of Arnhem, Holland, four miles west of Antwerp. This was a daylight mission as opposed to the early-morning or late-evening missions the men had taken part in months earlier. During this mission, telephone communication by lines strung along the tow rope between glider and plane was used. This was a new concept that allowed the pilot to pick up a phone to talk to the glider pilot, no longer relying on a light to indicate when the drop zone had been reached.

The scheduled drop of airborne paratroopers south of

the Arnhem Bridge was unsuccessful on September 18, the second day of the mission, because of bad weather. All gliders and C-47s of the 50th and 52nd Troop Carrier Wings had to return to base. After the initial Market-Garden missions, the job of the 50th TCS was to help resupply the men on the ground. Air evacuation of wounded belonged to the IX TCC. The weather did not cooperate in this effort. Airborne troops needed supplies, food, and ammunition; wounded needed evacuation and care. The resupply line stretched 250 miles from the Normandy coast. Despite the great need, the English fog often held the planes on the ground. Only airborne operations of the highest priority diverted the wings' attention away from the pressing logistical needs of the ground units. The TCS could transport most, but not all, of the needs of the ground units by air.

The German resistance was stronger than expected in Belgium, and gains were limited to a fifty-mile advance. In the end, Market-Garden was considered a failed mission, but the soldiers required supplies nevertheless.

A resupply mission was planned for September 25 because the weather forecast called for favorable conditions. The men of the 50th Troop Carrier Squadron were restricted to the base in anticipation that the mission would be a go. But that morning there was no field secured by the ground troops that the planes could land on.

By 1100 hours that morning, the airborne troops had pushed the Germans back a mile from a former German fighter field. It consisted of a rectangular dirt pasture of 1,000 yards by 1,400 yards. By 1115, the 50th squadron took off, hoping that the field would still remain in friendly hands by the time they arrived.

At 1350, the first C-47 landed on the dirt strip. The planes arrived in a long line. Pilots landed and immediately taxied to the side. There was no air traffic control and the landing pattern was jammed, but all planes landed safely. The unloading of each plane was accomplished as swiftly as possible.

Nearly one hundred C-47s on the field at one time was a tempting target for the Germans. American and British fighters flew overhead to keep the Luftwaffe away. The last C-47 took off to head back to base three hours later. One hundred thirty-two jeeps, seventy-three trailers, thirty-one motorcycles, 3,374 gallons of gasoline, 730 pounds of rations and ammo, and 882 men had all been delivered to the ground troops. The wounded and glider pilots were loaded and the planes left to find their way safety far behind the front lines. "Job well done," reported the group war diary. All of this was accomplished with full coverage by newspaper reporters, radio broadcasts, and photographers.

In October 1944, the intensity of the fighting caused a sharp rise in the number of battle-fatigue casualties among American troops. Psychiatric casualties from battle fatigue or shell shock were expected; the fear of being killed or maimed was as inevitable as gunshots or shrapnel wounds for the pilots and crews. Still, the number was troubling. General Eisenhower stated he was concerned about the men and this increasing problem. The condition often materialized because commanders liked to use well-proven troops instead of fresh, untried men to tackle key objectives. For instance, the same air force and paratroopers groups that participated in the invasion of Normandy lead the way in Operation Market-Garden.

One pilot described a horrible, persistent sense of guilt

after learning a plane had crashed with forty-two men aboard. He knew it was not his fault, but some part of him overrode that idea. He was consumed by fear, remorse, and apprehension. The terror of the unknown or misunderstood filled him with suffocating dread.

The stress and pressure on a pilot was enormous. He felt responsible for the thirty-two people aboard his plane and for even more men if he was flight-group or squadron leader on that mission. He had to make life-and-death decisions while traveling slowly, holding formation, and taking enemy fire. There was no armor on the planes or gliders, and rarely fighter plane protection on the serials. (The resupply missions were flown in serials, which involved a group of planes instead of the entire squadron. A serial was made of up of a number of aircraft, usually forty-five or more, dedicated to one particular delivery of supplies to a particular area.)

Captain Bob Jones, a TCC pilot, shared this comment about pilot fear: "Troop carrier combat missions in the C-47 were flown low and slow, often times towing fully loaded gliders that were very vulnerable to enemy ground fire in an aircraft originally built for commercial use with only a rear entrance to exit aircraft in emergency situations, okay for crew in cabin but near impossible for the pilots up front. With high aircraft losses this fear became a real mental problem for C-47 pilots."[1] On the other hand, bombers had protective armor and emergency exits built into the airframe for different crew stations, providing more successful bailout results.

One of Lamb's friends, Buck Buchanan, wrote a letter to

Lamb after the war recalling a fear that his plane would be lost while the 50th was stationed at Poix:

> I had a premonition that "son of the bitch" [Buck's plane, number 335] was going to get shot down, so I took a jeep and went to a B-17 base and got a load of flack suites [sic]. I worked until 2:30 installing those suites [sic] or vests in 335 behind the cockpit and companion way floors.
>
> Upon completion of this task [I] went to operations where "Smithy" advised me that I could relax now as I wasn't going on that last drop of the war, over the Rhine River.
>
> This upset me because if that plane was going to get shot down I wanted no other pilot to be driving it. "Can't help it Buck, you are officially on orders to train pilots in the new C-46."
>
> That premonition was so strong, I timed the mission and when I was sure they were on their way back I took the C-46 and flew back and forth by those C-47s three times. Only one plane missing—335. Three hours of non-stop flying under the conditions we experienced that day didn't leave much reserve energy.
>
> Next day we found all of the crew. Got aboard the C-46 with me doing the driving and we went up and picked up the plane's crew.

Buck's vision became a reality, establishing his unfortunate ability to foretell such tragedies. After D-Day, the pilots were ordered not to duck flak or take any evasive action if they came under fire. They were to remain on the instructed flight plan, making no change in course or altitude during a mission even if guns or artillery were in the area or shots were being fired.

More and more pilots and crewmen from Lamb's squadron had an opportunity to return home on leave and escape these horrors, albeit temporarily. Lamb, however, remained in France. On October 19, he wrote to his mother:

> The mail going both ways has been very slow lately. I've been feeling a little bad of late and am staying in sick quarters for a while 'til I feel better. Lots more of our personnel have recently gone back to the states, in fact, most of the fellows over 35 have gone back.
>
> You asked about needing Xmas present. I'd rather you wouldn't send any, because I think we might *accidentally* be on our way back by that time. I've told Betty so much about the possibility of returning before this that she will never believe I'm back 'til I walk in the front door. How does she look these days? I hope she is feeling well. I never knew that I could get so homesick as I am.
>
> Things look better everyday [*sic*] now, and this mess may terminate before very long. Thanks again for the offer of Xmas presents, but as I say, there may be a wild chance that I may be home by then. Keep your fingers crossed.
>
> I do routinely a small amount of writing now as compared to a year ago this time. That is true of most of us over here now. Time spent as we spend it tends to dull one's content of thought. We seldom do anything that is interesting to us even, much less to anyone at home.

Jaded, the men and planes of the 50th TCS continued to fly fresh provisions to the soldiers on the ground, including medical supplies, blood plasma, wire, clothing, PSP matting, "dudding" (for treating clothes against poison gas), tires, binoculars, .45 caliber pistols, vehicles, artillery, equipment, ammunitions, bazookas, back mortars, jerricans of gas, and food for the French people who were being liberated. The delivery process remained unchanged: C-47s pulled gliders and their loads of men and equipment. In October, the 50th TCS supplied over seventeen million pounds of freight to the front line, the most the squadron had hauled to date. In mid-October, they received a hurry-up call for supplies. Because of the freezing temperatures, anti-freeze for equipment was desperately needed at the front.

President Roosevelt was elected to a fourth term the following month, which brought in poor weather conditions for those men fighting in Europe. On November 23, twenty-three new pilots joined the 50th TCS. Eight freight missions were flown in November, delivering a total of 822,407 pounds of ammunition.

Lamb's time was spent treating severe yet commonplace colds. The ground troops fighting at the front had a difficult time enduring the snowy, below-freezing weather. Frostbite and trench foot became serious medical concerns. With heavy fighting in and around Metz, France, the hospitals overflowed with casualties. Over the course of the Battle of Metz, fifty evacuation flights transported wounded from the area; these were lifesaving flights for many of these men. The most seriously wounded soldiers were evacuated to the large hospital in Membury, England.

During the war, patients wounded in combat were taken from the front lines and treated through a chain of evacuation. Nearest to the battlefield were battalion aid stations, where surgeons, medics, and corpsmen performed lifesaving surgical procedures to stabilize the wounded. At collecting stations, "collecting companies would change bandages on incoming wounded, adjust splints, administer plasma, and combat shock while preparing the patient for the next step in the chain," a clearing station. Located four to six miles behind collecting stations, clearing stations triaged patients, treated less-life-threatening injuries, and transported wounded to field hospitals behind the front lines. After recuperating at a field hospital for a week or two, wounded were transferred to evacuation hospitals, "400-bed semi mobile facilities that were to be located approximately ten to fifteen miles behind the front lines." From there, patients were either sent back to the front or taken to a station hospital — which received "patients who needed a longer term than a field or evacuation hospital could provide, but less than 180 days" — or a general hospital — a non-mobile facility situated 70-100 miles from the front. While general hospitals were equipped for long-term care, patients were sent home to the United States if their recovery time exceeded six months.[2] Interestingly, though, during WWII, 95 percent of hospital admissions were non-combat related.

The Ninth Air Force was directed to equip all transport aircraft with litters and to give medical care and treatment to all casualties during flight and at airdromes. The patients were delivered as close as possible to a fixed hospital in England, and pilots were encouraged to return from the forward lines with patients. However, this depended on air superiority, the tactical situation, and the weather.

The process of evacuating wounded patients by air had its challenges, as Martin Wolfe describes in his book *Green Light*. For example, according to the military regulations, "patients with chest wounds were not supposed to fly above 3,000 feet; the thinner air up there made patients breathe harder. But complying often meant flying through low clouds and turbulent air, equally bad for wounded men." To avoid destabilizing patients, pilots could bank their planes at no more than a twenty degree angle when they carried litters. Of course, "this made for vexingly slow approaches to a landing field. Sometimes heated arguments on handling the plane would break out between nurse and pilot." But the most difficult aspect of evacuation missions was the unpleasant odor of gangrene that would fill the cabin of the planes. "Even today," a medical crewmen noted, "I have only to close my eyes and call up a memory of a med-evac mission, and the sensation of that overpowering, disgustingly sweet smell fills my head."[3]

Twelve litter patients or eighteen walking wounded constituted a planeload. Twenty-four wounded could be taken if there was no other choice. For most of the injured, this evacuation flight was their first time in an airplane. Unlike these men, the nurses were very comfortable and had experience flying in a C-47. Some had even been airline stewardesses before the war.

Transport and ground crews with little or no medical training often had emotional complications from handling severely wounded patients. One mechanic wrote: "Whenever they brought in the wounded some of us would go up on the flight line and help unload those fellows. A few of us, I remember couldn't handle that. . . . Some of these had arms gone, legs gone, the sides of their faces shot away, holes in their bellies and more of that sort of thing.

But somehow, I was able to cope with this; I helped unload many of those poor fellows into ambulances."[4] Usually rest away from the devastating job of seeing to the wounded helped. Personnel were sent to US recreational areas in Nice or to the Hotel Martinez in Cannes for R&R.

Thanksgiving 1944 was spent in dismally damp weather. A few officers stationed in France, mostly Air Force officers, had the special treat of being invited to enjoy a meal in a local French family's home for the holiday.

December saw no improvement in the fighting. Hitler launched a counteroffensive on December 16, 1944, in the Ardennes region of Belgium and Holland. His idea was to drive the Allies back to Antwerp and defeat the British 21st Army Group and the First and Ninth US Armies. Because of the poor weather, the Germans were able to surprise the Allies and made rapid gains. The penetration into Allied lines became known as the Battle of the Bulge.

The Allied troops on the ground were fighting in horribly cold weather and conditions that prohibited supplies from arriving. Part of the 50th TCS flew resupply missions to the troops in the Bastogne area of Belgium in mid-December.

On December 27, the IX TCC participated in Operation Repulse. The trooper carriers flew emergency resupply missions to the front with an intensified schedule, as the weather allowed, when they were not flying airborne missions. Delivering supplies to the surrounded troops in Bastogne meant avoiding heavy flak and navigating constantly moving gun emplacements, making for difficult missions.

Whenever the weather broke enough to fly, the urgency

of the situation allowed little time for air support to be arranged. The flight routes were still not much more than guesses because of the low visibility. Glider pilots often flew blind in the overcast weather. Parapacks filled the planes and gliders loaded with ammunition and gasoline were towed.

In the book *Green Light,* Jesse Coleman, a flight surgeon in the 81st TCS, remembered:

> After the Battle of the Bulge they ordered every Flight Surgeon off his own Field and to the nearest base hospital. . . . I was able to give about half of those guys passes for visiting some nearby city; but several of these never did come back to that hospital. They took off for the high country, and when I was ready to come back to Membury, three or four of them still had not returned![5]

During those weeks in December 1944, Lamb was aware of the difficult time the troops were having during the Battle of the Budge. Despite the freezing conditions, Lamb said he had no trouble staying warm where he was. He and his roommate shared a tent with a stove.

Lamb wrote home in December to let his family know that he had been on the continent a great deal and had enjoyed his time there. Lamb mentioned that he had hoped to send his sisters perfume from Paris. He had thought at one time he might be home in a few months, but he supposed those plans had fallen through. He requested they send him the National Geographic maps of the world — Europe, the Far East, and the Philippines — so he could keep up with how each of the fronts was doing.

Chapter Ten
Belgium and Germany

After being stationed in Poix for a couple of months, Lamb was sent to care for patients in rest camps in Belgium and Germany. He began his work in Belgium by evaluating injured men. On January 22, 1945, Lamb wrote to his brother and sister-in-law: "There isn't much new as usual from this end of the line. I have been in Belgium recently for a period of duty and will be returning again soon. The weather here is terrific; snow (10 inches), then rain and slush. This cycle takes place every week. If Uncle Joe Stalin keeps going maybe we won't have to worry about it much longer. Thanks again for the nice Christmas package you sent me. Everything was delicious, a rare treat, and greatly appreciated."

The main group of the 50th Troop Carrier Squadron moved from England to Poix, France, in February 1945, joining the crews already permanently stationed there. The March 1945 entry in the 50th War Diary documented that there were 150 officers and 293 enlisted in the squadron at that time.

In March 1945, the US Marines were fighting for the Japanese island of Iwo Jima in the Pacific, and halfway around the world the Allies in the European theater were crossing the Rhine in a push to move into the German homeland.

On March 24, the 50th TCS participated in Operation Varsity, the planned airborne assault over the Rhine River, once again dropping paratroopers and pulling gliders filled with paratroopers. Operation Varsity was a single phase of the larger mission Operation Plunder. The Allies had already taken bridges in two additional places further south. This mission established a hold on the northern section of the Rhine near Wesel, Germany, and closer to Berlin.

The 6th Airborne Division were veterans of the Normandy invasion, while the 17th Airborne were experiencing their first mission. Operation Varsity was the second biggest air drop of the war, Normandy being the largest. The mission was notable for having the most airborne dropped in one day.

W. B. Hertig, a pilot with the 50th Troop Carrier Squadron, had a unique experience during the mission that stayed with him long after the war ended:

> Our Group was the last group, our squadron was the last squadron, and I was the last plane—Tail End Charlie!
>
> The mission probably started around 8 a.m. and we didn't take off until late morning. Bingham "Dog" Wolles and me off his wing. Trombley was my crew chief. As we got further into the mission, we had to keep throttling back and throttling back because of the hundreds of planes and gliders ahead of us. To keep from stalling out, Bingham began making 360 degree large turns, which as you can guess caused the gliders to go way over the qualified speeds. After we made the 360, then we would go full throttle to catch up to the rest of the mission, only to have throttle back and throttle back and then do another 360. At the time, I didn't think about the speed the gliders must be going on those sharp turns, especially my glider, because we were last.

Needless to say our four planes made it back safely. A week or so later, the glider pilots started drifting back . . . I was sitting in my tent with my roomies, Harman, Karwood, North, and Gehrt, and we heard a lot of carousing and noise coming from another part of the squadron. The word was that the returning glider pilots, not finding any cognac available, had requisitioned some 150 proof alcohol from the medics and were mixing it with grapefruit juice. Pretty soon a glider pilot staggered into our tent—his name was McDonald and he looked to be about 6 feet, 5 inches and about 200 pounds.

He walked into the tent and said, "Where's Hertig?" I looked around and everyone was looking at me so I meekly raised my hand. He came over to me, eyes glazed and voice raised and said, "You're the worst damn pilot I've ever flown with." He let loose with a few more cuss words and staggered away.

Forty years later, I was at the Little Rock 50th Reunion and I heard he was going to arrive for the Saturday evening festivities. I kept asking if anyone had seen McDonald. Finally someone pointed him out to me. What a surprise! He was only about 6 feet tall and about 180 pounds. I walked up to him and said, "I'm Hertig," and stuck out my hand. He said, "You're still the worst damn pilot," and stuck out his hand and gave me a big bear hug. That was really a special time.

A month or so later he was out fishing and died in his boat. At least that's a lot better way to go than doing 360s in a glider over enemy territory!

This was the last glider drop ever made in combat, so we should be in the history books.[1]

Ground fire was heavy as the unarmed planes flew into Germany. The IX TCC encountered primarily rifles and light machine guns at first and then moved into heavy machine-gun fire and light cannons blazing. Gun towers were given a wide berth by the pilots. From the planes, the crew could hear the sounds of large guns. Smoke and flames were visible from burning vehicles and buildings. The all-pervasive smell of death filled the air, even at five hundred feet above ground. John Luthy's plane was hit by enemy fire on its way out of Poix during Operation Varsity. Before he reached his drop zone, "Flak rocked the plane and made quite a racket flying everywhere."

The left engine was hit and caught fire. We put it out with the one burst of carbon dioxide that we had. Almost immediately we were hit again, both in the companionway area and the left engine. The engine burst into flames and was vibrating the whole airplane. As we tried to feather the props the whole engine fell off the plane. With the sudden loss of the engine weight and the full power on the right engine, we started to roll over. We cut the power on the right engine and were able to roll out level, but it took both of us holding aileron and rudder to do so.

While this was going on, Gail and Quentin were near the side door at the rear of the aircraft with their parachutes on. They had been advised before we took off that if anything happened to the plane during the mission they were to do whatever they felt was right—not to wait for any formal instructions from us. We were told later by observers that both bailed out and landed safely just near the west bank of the Rhine River.

As the plane continued to burn, the cockpit became engulfed in thick black smoke so that it was impossible to see and tough to breath. We released the escape hatch in the roof, which helped to vent the smoke a great deal and we could then see enough to observe the instruments and see out of the plane. Just enough power was used from the right engine to keep flying while descending as quickly as we could. Visibility outside was terrible because of the smoke screen and things were moving and happening very fast.

At one point during this ordeal, we both considered leaving the plane through the escape hatch without a parachute (they were not in the cockpit and we only wore a harness), but thought better of it.

As we're descending very rapidly, suddenly out of the fog electric high tension transmission wires were right in front of us. We both hauled back on the control column and narrowly cleared the wires. We dropped the nose immediately and found a level garden patch of ground in front of us. We cut the power to make a belly landing, but just about that time the wheels touched down. We had not put the gear down but presumed they dropped down and locked when we were hit. We're on the ground now. Really moving, trying to stop this thing. We're both on the brakes, but with no hydraulics, no brakes. Here again, it seems something was always right in front of us. This time it's a two-story brick building and soldiers are bailing out of it. It was our good fortune that the plane stopped short of it.

The plane is fully engulfed in flames just behind us and the escape hatch is the only way out. Bob [Heinemann] exited first and jumped to the ground with his flak suit on, injuring his leg. I followed him, but released my flak suit first and had no injury.

As we hobbled away from the plane toward the building, we were greeted by soldiers with an Australian accent. They gave us tea and crackers and drove us to a Field some distance away. I believe they assisted Bob in getting him to a medical facility where his leg was treated.[2]

Later that month, a press release was circulated sharing the details of Luthy and Bob Heinemann's experience. It identified the 50th Troop Carrier Squadron as "one of the most successful squadrons of the U.S. Troop Carrier Forces."[3]

With Varsity completed and the Allied troops pressing toward Berlin, the troop carrier command's job turned to flying resupply missions to the front when weather permitted. Gasoline, ammunition, and food were not easily obtained other than by plane. In April 1945, the 50th TCS was cited for outstanding achievement for their work in delivering supplies, rations, ammunition, and important freight to the front lines.

Non-battle casualties for the month of April exceeded the total of all previous battle and non-battle casualties since the arrival of the 50th TCS to the European theater in May 1943. Thirty-six freight missions were flown, hauling 1,745,206 pounds of freight. The 50th TCS also transported more than two thousand passengers to various points on the continent.

On April 12, 1945, a midnight radio news broadcast announced the death of President Roosevelt. A memorial service was held for the president at Headquarters.

Lamb remained assigned to the Poix field with the 50th TCS but was loaned to other units until two months before the end of the war. At the time of the president's death in April, he was assigned to a rest camp in Germany.

Throughout the spring, the 50th Troop Carrier Squadron continued to carry out regular missions between England and France ferrying men, wounded, and supplies. This type of work brought unusual mechanical problems for the

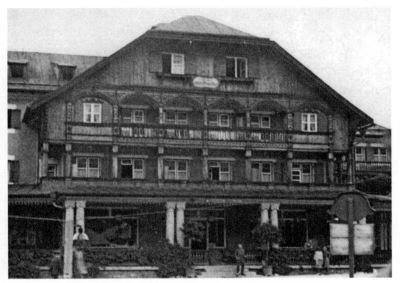

Bavarian hotel used for R&R in Germany

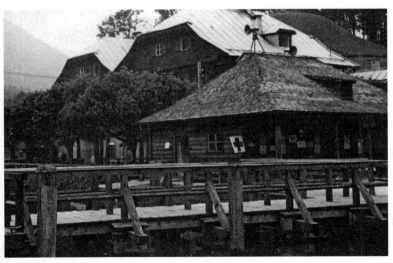

Dispensary at a rest camp in Germany

planes. For the first time since Sicily, it became necessary to ground planes because of flat tires. The increased incidence of flat tires was due to the large numbers of sharp rocks and pieces of shrapnel on the captured runways, which were mostly dirt or sod. There were likewise a larger number of engine changes because of the increased number of hours the planes were flying to evacuate wounded.

The 50th TCS War Diary offered some detail on the loss the squadron had suffered in this area:

> The enormous tonnage of freight hauled during the month was not without its cost in planes and lives within the unit. Since coming overseas the 50th had never had a flying non-battle casualty in almost two years of overseas service until 6 April 1945. On that day, five aircraft were involved in two accidents, separated in distance by about 85 miles and in time, by about 20 minutes in which nine officers and six enlisted men were killed. Two days later an enlisted man walked into the moving propeller of a C-109 and died two-and one half hours later, making the unprecedented total of sixteen non-battle casualties for the month of April.[4]

During the same month, seven new planes arrived to replace those destroyed during the crashes. This increased the squadron's aircraft strength considerably.

In a letter dated April 4, 1945, Betty Myhr wrote to her mother-in-law: "I've not heard from Lamb beyond Jan. 9th. Have you? Maybe he's on his way home! All my brothers are alright. Things look very good right now and perhaps it will all be over sooner than we think."

Chapter Eleven
Combat Control Team

In the April 1945 entry into the 50th War Diary, it was recorded that Capt. Lamb B. Myhr, Squadron Flight Surgeon, and Cpl. Howard Bloomfied were assigned to the DS (Detached Service) with Control Team No. 2, B-86, by Wing Special Order. Combat Control Teams provided forward treatment for patients during combat operations. Winning battles required the rapid return of temporarily disabled soldiers to their units. These forward units provided consultation, triage, immediate treatment, and mental-health evaluations. The control team's primary mission was to swiftly return men to combat.

Lamb's job also consisted of changing bandages on incoming wounded, adjusting splints, administering plasma, and treating combat shock while preparing patients to be moved to rear hospitals. Because the front lines were fluid, control teams moved between airfields, working quickly to secure the fields and move causalities behind the front lines to medical care. Being near the front meant Lamb was in danger regularly. Lamb described his new assignment to his brother in a letter dated April 10, 1945:

> I'm mailing you a few packages in a few weeks. They are
> German rifles, brand new, never been fired — that I recently

217

obtained in the drive. I've been on detached service with a control unit which operates Fields as soon as they are captured. It's a good job and very interesting. I handle the air evacuation of wounded and anything else that comes up. I crossed the Rhine in a glider on the recent move. The German people are a defeated, bewildered lot and from the looks of things they won't try it again 20 years from now. We are really rolling these days. Last place I hit there was still food on the table — we caught them eating lunch! I have a Mercedes-Benz sedan and big Jerry motorcycle for private transportation (what a life!) Also lot of captured cognac is available. I can send you several rifles as I have only a dozen. I'll send them as soon as I get back to a home base (2-3 weeks maybe.)

A memorandum from IX Troop Carrier Command Headquarters issued on April 5, 1945, established the reasoning and guidelines for the newly formed Combat

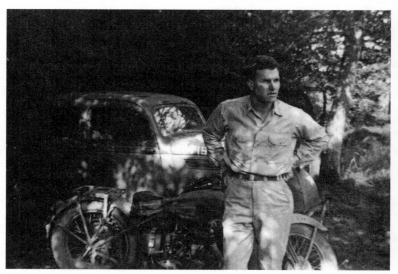

Lamb with his "private transportation"

Control Teams. During Operations Neptune and Market-Garden, a number of problems with rapid appraisal and the need for necessary action had arisen. Those happened during different phases of the supply delivery and the resupply by glider and parachute. The trouble was the changing battle lines that often resulted in the landing zone (LZ) and delivery zone (DZ) being occupied by enemy forces when resupply or reinforcement was scheduled to the tactical area.

Because of this issue, leadership decided that eight Combat Control Teams should be formed, two each for the 82nd, 101st, 17th, and 13th Airborne Divisions of the XVIII Corps (Airborne). Each Control Team consisted of two units, complete in and of themselves, that were able to operate individually. This concept was absolutely essential to providing reliable communications and allowed for a complete unit to be carried in one glider, preventing scattering when two gliders could not land in the same zone. An extra unit also permitted reshuffling of personnel and equipment, providing communication in a minimum amount of time. In order to provide two complete units for each Combat Control Team, additional aircraft and gliders were required. This demand doubled the number of glider pilots and C-47 pilots needed for each airborne mission.

Combat Control Teams were responsible for four primary functions: 1) to establish themselves with XVIII Corps (Airborne) Headquarters and coordinate all outgoing messages through the corps or division commander; 2) to coordinate with the Corps G-3 (an Army division); 3) to arrange glider pick-up from combat landing zones in emergency situations; and 4) to establish radio contact with IX Troop Carrier Command and First Allied Airborne Army Headquarters to facilitate the transmission of information, such as weather reports.

The data transmitted by the Combat Control Teams helped remove previously unknown threats to airborne missions and was extremely valuable in keeping those missions running smoothly. The IX Troop Carrier Command was now regularly informed of the following: known strength of points of resistance that could jeopardize certain drop zones and landing zones; hazards in glider landing zones and recommendations for eliminating those hazards, if possible; recommended relocation of glider landing zones; and recommended relocation of resupply drop zones. Through the work of Combat Control Teams, the IX Troop Carrier Command also benefited from better contact with incoming Troop Carrier Serial Leaders and, when possible, were privy to messages relative to the concentration of enemy troops and enemy air activity.

These Troop Carrier Combat Control Teams were specially equipped and trained to properly perform their duties under any conditions. Essentially, they were like the air support parties organized to support the airborne corps and divisions. Their formation, development, and operation was based significantly on the experiences gained and lessons learned from previous airborne operations of the war.

Personnel were given special training in how to handle themselves properly under any condition they might encounter, which was essential in preventing high casualty rates. It was necessary that they qualify as infantrymen, so the air-support personnel trained with the airborne units they supported. This training included lessons in the use of radio and cryptographic equipment.

Each Combat Control Team consisted of one glider pilot with a minimum of five hundred hours in a powered plane, participation in two combat missions, and service as a flying control operator; three glider pilots with radio operator qualifications (who would be used as both glider pilots and radio operators); and one radio operator who could also double as a mechanic. All personnel were qualified to drive a jeep pulling a trailer.

These men were assigned specific equipment necessary to perform their listed duties. Required for each team were two jeeps, one a specialized one-fourth-ton jeep with a rebuilt body that provided adequate space for both equipment — including a generator — and an operator to efficiently man a mounted radio; one SCR-399 or SCR-499 radio with a PE-75 power unit; and one VHF radio. Also included in the setup was a noiseless, portable typewriter and three M-209 portable cipher converters. (To communicate securely, the Allies would establish codes that would change every thirty-two hours. These codes were transmitted over a certain frequency; the M-209 was used to decipher the code and send messages in turn.)

Both the SCR-399 and SCR-499 were mobile, high-powered Signal Corps Radios that could transmit communication while stationary or while moving on a rough road at high speed. The power plant for the radio was mounted in the trailer that was towed behind the jeep. If necessary, the SCR could be remotely controlled from up to one mile away. The VHF (very high frequency) radio added less than 100 pounds to the total load and fit into the available space. VHF radios afforded an auxiliary channel of communication to aircraft in flight and were mounted in the jeeps to provide greater dispersion of equipment. The supply of auxiliary power equipment for each jeep was critical yet difficult to procure.

In addition to this particular equipment, Combat Control Teams carried a variety of documents, including a special code (similar to an air support request code) necessary to deciphering messages; a ground-authentication code; and a point-to-point authentication code.

As the war continued, troops spread farther from England, from where the generals were directing the Allies. This distance made reliance on direct contact between the Combat Control Teams and Troop Carrier Command Headquarters impossible. In response, relay stations were used to ensure contact. Serving as an intermediary between Headquarters and the teams, these stations were located on the front lines closer to the Combat Control Teams than to the Troop Carrier Command Headquarters. One of the eight teams could be used as the relay station: If the distance was too far to get a clear message, one team set up a position while another would move ahead. The message would be transmitted to the relay station, which would then pass it on to another unit or to headquarters. These were flexible, mobile units. Avoiding communication breakdowns was paramount since the front lines were changing so quickly.

Troop Carrier Combat Teams No. 1 and No. 2 were placed on detached service with XVIII Corps (Airborne) for five days, effective March 12, 1945. This provided the necessary amount of time for the teams to get acquainted with the units they would operate alongside. The teams were first deployed during Operation Varsity, accompanying the XVIII Corps (Airborne). Normally two gliders were needed per team, but to transport all personnel and equipment two additional gliders were required. Special pick-up equipment was also needed.

The senior officers of Combat Control Team No. 2, of which Lamb became a member, offered a report of their mission in Operation Varsity, which took place on March 24, 1945. After the briefings were completed and the six gliders were loaded, the pilots took off for their landing zones. According to the report, "all six gliders landed in LZ N, three at one end of the LZ, and three at the other end."

> The party was under small arms fire during the landing and for about one hour after landing. The glider infantry consolidated the LZ area before unloading their gliders. The Control Teams took cover in the woods by previous agreement with the glider infantry until they started unloading. . . . It is a very good idea for the Control Teams to go into the LZ first, as they have a better chance of landing personnel and equipment in an operating condition.
>
> The two Control Teams did not contact each other until 1800 hours. No attempt had been made to transmit at LZs. Both Teams arrived at the Division CP [command post] at 1700 hours, and reported to Colonel Messinger, G-3. A message was sent to Troop Carrier Command headquarters that both Teams and equipment were intact."[1]

By the spring of 1945, the letters from Lamb began arriving to his family with an actual location on them as opposed to the notation of "somewhere in Europe." In the past, he had been required to send blind letters hiding the location of the combat zone he was in. He wrote from Central Germany on April 14, 1945:

> I hope and believe that the war in this section will be over by the time this letter reaches you. I've been in a different job for the past few weeks. I am with a team that surprises Fields as soon as they are taken. We have really been moving fast lately. To get an idea where I might be and how fast I'm moving, I was in Kassel about 2 weeks ago. Have found this job very interesting. I take care of the air evacuation of wounded from the front-line hospitals. The lines move so fast now that it's hard to keep up with them. Things are very encouraging. The German people are completely beaten in some areas, but others are not so. I have gotten a few nice souvenirs including $1200 camera which I hope to bring back. I've had no word from you or Betty for 6 1/2 weeks.
>
> Lot of love, write soon,

All Troop Carrier Combat Control Teams were being used as field control parties at forward fields in Germany. They were highly useful in this type of work due to their extreme mobility, a prerequisite because the battle front was moving forward so rapidly. Fields were soon too far behind the scene of action to be useful for resupply operations.

During the first twenty days of April 1945, 35,962 wounded were evacuated from battle areas. On April 5, the 50th Troop Carrier Squadron delivered more tonnage in one day than they had through the first three months of 1945 combined. Ground travel was difficult; the successful air bombing caused so much damage that the only way to move a great distance was by plane. For the first time, general hospitals were able to operate three hundred miles behind the front line.

A little more than a month later, Lamb wrote his mother again, this time from Austria. His letter was written on May 17 on a German's personalized stationery, demonstrating both that the Germans' personal lives were equally disrupted by the war and that American troops would use whatever material they could find to send news back home to their loved ones.

> I have been moving around so much lately that I haven't written very much to anyone. Have been working in Germany, Austria, Czechoslovakia, and spent one day in Copenhagen, Denmark. The part of Germany around Munich, where I have spent most of the time, is one of the most beautiful spots I have ever seen. All the mountains in this part of Austria are now snow-capped and truly beautiful. The "control team" that I'm on has been getting out Frenchmen and Belgians from airports in this area. They have been slave labor in Germany during the war, some prisoners in concentration camps. I recently visited the concentration camp at Dachau, near Munich, and it was hard to believe my own eyes. Buchenwald and Weimar are the same way. I actually don't believe the average German citizen knew all that was carried on by the SS and Gestapo. Some of the towns over here are completely destroyed, some untouched. Munich, Aachen, Duren, Nurnberg have been almost leveled by bombing alone. I am thankful that our country was never bombed, but believe it would be necessary to make some people realize a war existed.

> Yes, I had heard of Pat Fowlkes being killed. He was a fine man; never have I seen a man who was better liked by everyone. I am sorry for his wife and children.

News from you and Betty comes very seldom, because it has to be flown to me here from the base in France and I receive some every 10 days or so. My chances of coming home within the next 3-4 months are very good. And when I do come, I will not be sent on to the Pacific, because anyone who was in the African campaign will not have to go to the Pacific (they say).

I will be taking a trip to Oslo in the next 4 days for one day only. I'm going on a plane after some Americans who were in the hospitals there after having been shot down several months ago.

Take care of yourself. I love and miss you,

Chaplain Pat Fowlkes, Lamb's friend, had parachuted during a mission along with the soldiers he ministered to. He landed in a tree. The men worked to free him from the limbs, not realizing he'd been shot and was already dead. He was twenty-eight years old, with a wife and newborn baby. More than sixty years later, when Lamb told the story of the death of his friend, tears filled his eyes. Chaplains were not required to jump; when asked why Pat had, Lamb responded, "He thought he should be with his men."

In addition to seeing to the military wounded, Lamb spent time treating civilians who had been liberated from concentration camps. He'd been informed of the camps and their atrocities before he had to enter one for the first time. Because the work was so difficult emotionally, the doctors would rotate, each taking a three-day shift. Lamb attended the prisoners in Buchenwald, Dachau, and Weimar. Along with the other doctors, he helped determine who was healthy enough to be transferred to rest camps.

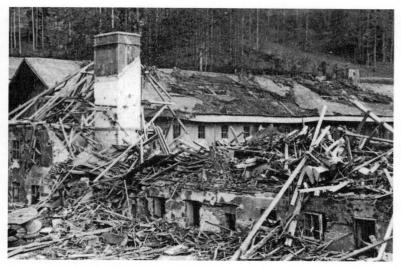

Bavarian building destroyed by a bombing

Buchenwald was located on the Ettersburg Mountain near Weimar, Germany, in the forested area of east-central Germany. Built in 1937, it was one of the first and largest concentration camps on German soil. Most detainees were political prisoners who comprised the work force for the local armament factories. Many men died from overwork, torture, beatings, and starvation. The road leading up Ettersburg Mountain was called Blood Street, a reference to the one thousand men who died building it. It was a huge concentration camp with eighty-eight sub-camps or external commandos that housed the work teams for the armament plants. Buchenwald was liberated on April 11, 1945, by US troops. There were twenty-one thousand prisoners housed in the camp at that time.

The home of Goethe, Schiller, Liszt, and Bach, the town of

Weimar was famous for its cultural life. By the time Lamb arrived, it had been almost completely obliterated from bombings. US soldiers forced the local townspeople to help clean up the dead bodies at Buchenwald.

Dachau was the first concentration camp established by the Nazis. Located on German soil near Munich in beautiful Bavaria, it had thirty sub-camps. Like Buchenwald, its political prisoners provided slave labor to the surrounding armament factories. When US troops liberated the camp on April 28, 1945, they found thirty railcars filled with dead bodies that the Nazis had not had time to dispose of before the Allies' arrival. Above the main gate of the camp read the words "Arbeit macht frei," meaning "Work makes you free."

Soon after liberation of the concentration camps, the 116th and 127th Evacuation Hospitals arrived in the area with

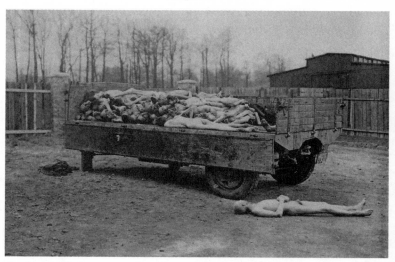

Buchenwald Concentration Camp (Courtesy National Archives and Records Administration)

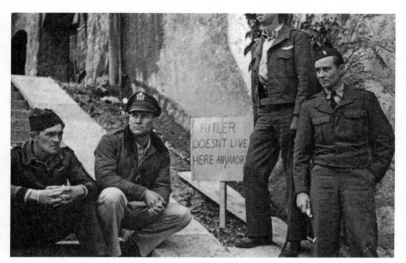

Lamb (second from left) at Hilter's "Eagles Nest"

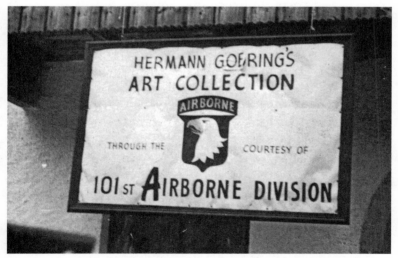

Sign posted in a village at the bottom of the mountain from Hitler's "Eagle's Nest"

food and medical supplies. Typhus, frozen feet, gangrene, bed sores, lice, and severe dermatitis were just a few of the medical difficulties plaguing the camps' survivors. Eight out of ten prisoners had tuberculosis, and many had neglected wounds inflicted by systematic torture. The majority of the survivors were weak from malnourishment; they were fed a thin beef mixture, skim milk, and a rice-and-sugar-based blend, but most had too fragile a digestive system to tolerate anything in their stomachs. Large numbers required special care, including constant reassurance that they would be taken care of and that they would live.

In April, Lamb learned through a radio broadcast that President Roosevelt had died and that Vice Pres. Harry Truman had become president. That same month, the IX Troop Carrier Command was officially removed from combat and spent an enormous amount of time returning liberated prisoners to their home countries. Flight surgeons continued to administer routine shots. Entire stations received a tetanus shot one month and typhus the next. They flew on single missions when available. The 314th Troop Carrier Group was cited for British battle honours for "outstanding performance of duty" for their work during the Normandy invasion.

During that spring, the Army Air Force surveyed 2,600 AAF combat veterans, both officers and enlisted men, who were returning from all overseas theaters. Seventy-two percent were favorably impressed with their squadron flight surgeon while only eighteen percent said they were dissatisfied with their flight surgeon's care.

Chapter Twelve
End of War

In May 1945, Lamb was still stationed in Germany, sharing a tent with a roommate. In the Pacific, the Japanese were being pushed back to their mainland by the US military. On the European front, a news bulletin announced that all Axis land, sea, and air forces in Italy surrendered unconditionally to Field Marshal Harold Alexander on May 2, 1945.

Lamb knew from talk around camp that the war was over four or five days before it was officially announced. Germany's unconditional surrender was signed at Reims at 0400 hours on May 7, 1945. On May 8, the 50th TCS flew demonstration flights over prisoner of war camps. Prime Minister Churchill officially announced Victory in Europe Day (VE Day) in a broadcast at 1300 hours Greenwich Mean Time (GMT) on May 8. The surrender became effective at 0001 hours on May 9, 1945. The occasion was marked in the 50th TCS's war dairy, which read as follows:

> The month of May saw the completion of two years of overseas services for the 50th Troop Carrier Squadron. The Squadron Air Echelon departed from the United States on 6 May 1943, and the Ground Echelon departed on 13 May 1943. The most significant happening of the month was receiving of a teletype message early on the morning of 7 May that terms of unconditional surrender had been signed

on behalf of the German High Command. The squadron took the news in stride and there was actually very little celebrating, the real celebration being reserved for the time when Japan capitulates.[1]

World War II was officially over in Europe; now the United States turned its full attention to the Japanese front.

All ground personnel were given physical examinations to determine their "physical profile." Shortly after Germany's surrender, a point system for rotation was announced that would determine whether personnel of the squadron would be sent to the Pacific. A man received one point for every month in uniform, one for each month overseas, five for each major campaign he participated in, five for each combat decoration, and twelve for each child up to three children. Any personnel with eighty-five points or more would be discharged in lieu of assignment in Japan. The system created much interest and speculation within the 50th TCS. When the points were awarded, 50 percent of the squadron personnel qualified to return stateside. Many of the remaining 50 percent had just fallen short of the required eighty-five points. They were involved in multiple campaigns, they had received medals, and yet they were being sent to the war in the Pacific instead of the safety of their homes.

Lamb had accrued more than one hundred points. He had been in uniform for three years, had been overseas for twenty-four months, had participated in three major campaigns, had received no fewer than three medals, and had one child. He was going home.

With the arrival of VE Day, many air force pilots were

already on their way home because they met mission-based requirements, a different system that sent pilots stateside when once they flew a certain number of missions. When they arrived, they were deactivated and returned to civilian life.

The men of the 50th TCS still stationed at Poix, France, had the opportunity to attend regular dances and parties and were given leave. Church services were held for all denominations. On May 12, 1945, seven C-47s were assigned to the squadron; this brought the total number of aircraft to twenty-nine — including an L-4 cub — and increased the number of officers on staff to seventy-nine. On May 13, the Ground Echelon celebrated its second anniversary of overseas service. Two years earlier on the same date they had landed at Casablanca.

During the month of May, all men of the 50th TCS were required to attend the showing of the film *Two Down and One to Go*, a reminder that the war was not over in the Pacific. At the same time, however, the men in the European theater experienced a relieving sense that the war was over. The general censorship of letters was discontinued, and June 6, 1945, was even "declared an army holiday as first anniversary of [the] D-Day landing." Personnel enjoyed "sightseeing trips over landing beaches and a party held in the evening in the mess hall."[2] Monthly individual press releases to a pilot or crew member's hometown paper were prepared; most included the same wording about a mission with a change in personal information. Their duties also changed, as in May the 50th TCS delivered 8,000 pounds of mail on just one run, handled personal luggage, transported prisoners of war, delivered medical supplies, and ferried upper echelon personnel and occupying forces.

By the end of the war, the IX Troop Carrier Command had flown more than 16,000 sorties, many in harm's way. The command had used 240 airfields, from Cherbourg to Leipzig. From airstrips across Germany, 451,000 American, British, French, Russian, Polish, African, Palestinian, Dutch, and Italian prisoners were returned home from their captivity. In 1945, the IX TCC delivered 44,212,200 tons of freight and 7,727,075 gallons of gas to the moving ground forces. The number of prisoners of war the command repatriated in the European Theater exceeded 69,000 in April and 184,000 in May. In June, the number dropped significantly to around 20,000. The 819th Medical Air Evacuation Squadron, which Lamb was assigned to in May 1945, issued a monthly evacuation report on May 31 that included statistical data such as average patient load per plane (29.5), maximum number of patients evacuated in any one plane (29), maximum number of patients evacuated in any one day (496), maximum altitude at which patients were flown (8,000 ft.), number of patients requiring oxygen (0), number of patients requiring intravenous therapy (0), and patient hours at altitude (over 10,000 ft.) (0).[3] Statistics about the wounded were further broken down into the number of patients on litters, the number of ambulant patients, the number of sick, the number of wounded, the injuries sustained, and where each man was from (Britain, France, Belgium, prisoner of war, or other). Burns, spinal injuries, and trench foot were common medical problems noted.

In a position of "military affluence," the 50th TCS force had wanted for little during the war. The only serious shortage they experienced was self-sealing tanks for planes. Minor inconveniences were the lack of watches, sunglasses, and penicillin for enlisted VD care. Officers of the Army Air Forces were considered well-educated and well-trained — and therefore well-paid. Lamb did not have to look far to find others less fortunate, such as the British, French, and German civilians.

June to late 1945 was spent downsizing the 50th TCS. Men were sent home by the hundreds, personnel were transferred, and the 50th Troop Carrier Squadron was moved under the responsibility of different wings, which lead to changes in its headquarters. New officers were taking over every two to three months. By December, the 50th TCS had shrunk to just two men, and on February 15, 1946, the war diary reads that no personnel and no equipment remained in Villacoublay, France, the current IX TCC headquarters.

One American soldier offered the reason a man goes to war: "You fight for the love and respect of the man next to you. You talk about love of country and hatred of the enemy but you fight for the buddy next to you."[4] During WWII, the Army Air Forces lost more men than any branch of service. Fifty percent of the men who joined died, which was more than the losses of all the other branches combined.

In July, the 50th TCS war diary includes a notation that Cap. Lamb B. Myhr had been replaced because he had been sent to the Zone of Interior in June to return to the United States. Lamb visited Normandy before leaving Europe. He then departed from Le Havre, France, by ship rather than plane, what he believed was the safer way to travel.

After five days on board, Lamb arrived in New York City.

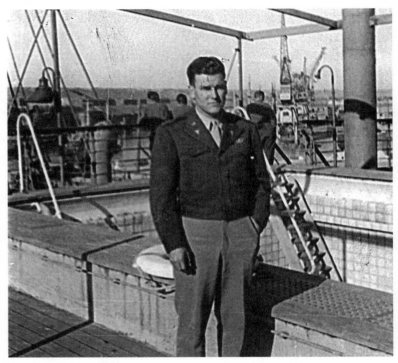

Lamb sailing home

From New York, he traveled by train to Atlanta, Georgia, where his wife, Betty, was there to meet him. He had already arrived in the States by the time the atom bomb was dropped in August 1945, which brought about the surrender of the Japanese in the Pacific and ended the war.

On December 24, 1945, Lamb permanently returned to Nashville after being discharged at the rank of major from the Army Air Forces in Atlanta. He went home to the house on East Clayton in Nashville where Betty and Bo, his son, lived while Lamb was overseas.

Many decorations and awards appear on Lamb's service record: European-African-Middle Eastern Campaign Medal with one silver service star; two Bronze Service Stars; Bronze Star Medal; Distinguished Unit Citation with one oak leaf cluster; World War II Honorable Service Lapel Button; World War II Victory Medal; and the American Campaign Medal.

The European-African-Middle Eastern Campaign Medal was given for personal service in all theaters between December 7, 1942, and November 8, 1945; it was the third-highest award given to a participant in that campaign. The Bronze Star, the fourth-highest combat award of the US Armed Forces, was awarded for heroic or meritorious achievement or service. Lamb received the Victory Medal as military personnel who served between December 7, 1941, and December 31, 1946; the Honorable Service Lapel Button for honorable service during the war; and the American Campaign Medal for air combat participation between December 7, 1941, and September 2, 1945.

Soon after returning to Nashville Lamb began his residency training in internal medicine at Vanderbilt Hospital and later at Thayer Hospital in Birmingham, Alabama. He became board-certified in internal medicine in 1948. In 1949, Lamb moved his family to Jackson, Tennessee, where he partnered with another physician and established the Jackson Clinic, which opened in 1950.

While Lamb didn't have trouble adjusting to life back home, his son, Bo, had trouble adjusting to having Lamb around. Bo was two-and-a-half weeks old when Lamb left for Europe, and Lamb had been gone for over two years.

Lamb told this story of his first morning at home after he returned from Europe: "Betty and I were still in bed. Bo came into the bedroom carrying a large picture book. He started hitting me on the head with the book and saying, 'You get out of my mother's bed.' I turned to Betty and said, 'Why didn't you tell this boy I'm his father?'" In 2007, Lamb's blue eyes twinkled when he looked at Betty and told that story. Lamb went on to father two more sons, David and

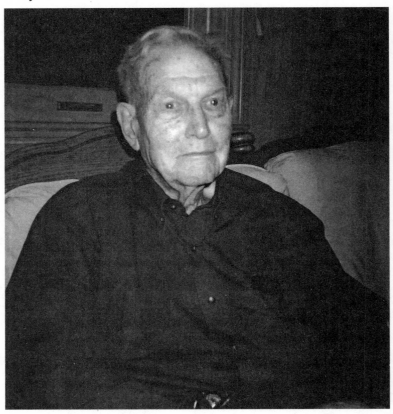

Lamb Myhr, age eighty-nine

Steve. He and Betty were married for more than sixty years.

When asked what life in the Army Air Forces had taught him, he responded, "How to be in the Army, but very little medicine. I learned map reading, army bed making, and to read markings." After a pause he added, "I learned to be careful." He reflected on the war with composure and realism: "I did what had to be done," he stated. "Everyone had a part. Freedom doesn't come without cost."

Lamb never revisited the places he had been during the war. When the 50th Troop Carrier Squadron had their reunion in Belgium, he did return to the area.

In 2005, thirteen members of the 50th TCS were still living. On April 16, 2008, Lamb died at his home while walking in the yard just three weeks before his ninety-first birthday.

Notes

Chapter One

1. Martin Wolfe, *Green Light!: A Troop Carrier Squadron's War From Normandy to the Rhine* (University of Pennsylvania Press, 1989; repr., Washington, DC: Center for Air Force History, 1993), 6.

2. "August 1943," in "50th Troop Carrier Squadron War Diary," including "Squadron Medical Journal" (unpublished manuscript, 1941-1945), accessed via Air Force Historical Research Agency, Maxwell Air Force Base, Montgomery, Alabama.

Chapter Two

1. Kenn C Rust, *The 9th Air Force in World II* (Falbrook, CA: Aero Publishers, 1967), 13.

2. "June 1943," in "50th Troop Carrier Squadron War Diary," including "Squadron Medical Journal" (unpublished manuscript, 1941-1945), accessed via Air Force Historical Research Agency, Maxwell Air Force Base, Montgomery, Alabama.

3. Ibid.

4. Robert G. Bramble, *History of the 50th Troop Carrier Squadron, 314th Troop Carrier Group, World War II.* Complied by a group historian, assembled, and audited.

5. Ernie Pyle, *Brave Men* (New York: Grosset & Dunlop, 1943), 168.
6. Cate, J. L. and W. F. Craven, eds., *The Army Air Forces in WWII* (HyperWar Foundation, 2011), 7:404, http://www.ibiblio.org/hyperwar/AAF/VII/AAF-VII-13.html. This log is a compilation that has been created from various sources to appear in *The Army Air Forces in WWII*.

Chapter Three
1. Ernie Pyle, *Brave Men* (New York: Grosset & Dunlop, 1943), 285.

Chapter Four
1. Robert G. Bramble, *History of the 50th Troop Carrier Squadron, 314th Troop Carrier Group, World War II*. Complied by a group historian, assembled, and audited.
2. Samuel T. Moore, with James Edwin Alexander, *Flight Surgeon: With the 81st Fighter Group in WWII* (Oklahoma City: Macedon), 1999. 156-57.
3. "December 1943," in "50th Troop Carrier Squadron War Diary," including "Squadron Medical Journal" (unpublished manuscript, 1941-1945), accessed via Air Force Historical Research Agency, Maxwell Air Force Base, Montgomery, Alabama.

Chapter Five
1. Ernest Gaillard, Jr., ed. and comp. William N. Gaillard, *Flight Surgeon: Complete and Unabridged Combat Medical*

Diary, US Eighth Army Air Forces, 381st Bomb Group, 242nd Medical Dispensary, Station 167 (Bloomington, IN: 1st Books Library, 2003) 69.

2. Ernie Pyle, *Brave Men* (New York: Grosset & Dunlop, 1943), 223.

Chapter Six

1. Martin Wolfe, *Green Light!: A Troop Carrier Squadron's War From Normandy to the Rhine* (University of Pennsylvania Press, 1989; repr., Washington, DC: Center for Air Force History, 1993), 214.

2. "May 1944," in "50th Troop Carrier Squadron War Diary," including "Squadron Medical Journal" (unpublished manuscript, 1941-1945), accessed via Air Force Historical Research Agency, Maxwell Air Force Base, Montgomery, Alabama.

3. James S. Nanney, "Aeromedical Challenges in Mounting an Attack From Great Britain," in "Army Air Forces Medical Services in World War II" (Air Force History and Museums Program, 1998), accessed April 8, 2005. http://www.afhso.af.mil/shared/media/document/AFD-100923-014.pdf.

4. "July 1943," in "50th Troop Carrier Squadron War Diary," including "Squadron Medical Journal" (unpublished manuscript, 1941-1945), accessed via Air Force Historical Research Agency, Maxwell Air Force Base, Montgomery, Alabama.

5. *Wartime Airfield Accidents*, WW2Talk, accessed April 10, 2005, http://ww2talk.com/forums/topic/20012-wartime-airfield-accidents.

6. Samuel T. Moore, with James Edwin Alexander, *Flight Surgeon: With the 81st Fighter Group in WWII* (Oklahoma City: Macedon Production Company, 1999), 84.

Chapter Seven

1. Samuel T. Moore, with James Edwin Alexander, *Flight Surgeon: With the 81st Fighter Group in WWII* (Oklahoma City: Macedon Production Company, 1999), 151.
2. Sid Dunagan, letter to Lamb Myhr.
3. Ammerman, Gale R. *An American Glider Pilot's Story: 81st Troop Carrier Squadron, 436th Troop Carrier Group*, Bennington, Vermont: Merriam Press, 2001. Page 16.

Chapter Eight

1. Joseph Harkeiwicz, "Daily Chronicles of a USAAF Unit in England for the Invasion of Europe," ed. by Lewis E. Johnston, from *We Are the 29th!: Troop Carrier Squadron- WWII*, accessed March 6, 2005 via the Air Mobility Command Museum, http://www.amcmuseum.org/history/wwii/daily_chronicles.php.
2. Ibid.
3. Robert G. Bramble, *History of the 50th Troop Carrier Squadron, 314th Troop Carrier Group, World War II*. Complied by a group historian, assembled, and audited.
4. Ernie Pyle, *Brave Men* (New York: Grosset & Dunlop, 1943), 244.

5. Bramble, *History of the 50th Troop Carrier Squadron*.

6. Gale R. Ammerman, *An American Glider Pilot's Story: 81st Troop Carrier Squadron, 436th Troop Carrier Group* (Bennington, Vermont: Merriam Press, 2001), 115.

7. Bramble, *History of the 50th Troop Carrier Squadron*.

8. Ibid.

9. Pyle, *Brave Men*, 347.

10. Ammerman, *An American Glider Pilot's Story*, 100.

Chapter Nine

1. Bob Jones, conversation with the author.

2. Evelyn Monahan and Rosemary Neidel-Greenlee, *And If I Perish: Frontline U.S. Army Nurses in World War II* (New York: Alfred A. Knopf, 2003), 29-30.

3. Martin Wolfe, *Green Light!: A Troop Carrier Squadron's War From Normandy to the Rhine* (University of Pennsylvania Press, 1989; repr., Washington, DC: Center for Air Force History, 1993), 419-20.

4. Ibid., 417.

5. Ibid., 355.

Chapter Ten

1. Robert G. Bramble, *History of the 50th Troop Carrier Squadron, 314th Troop Carrier Group, World War II*. Complied by a group historian, assembled, and audited.

2. Ibid.

3. "March 1945," in "50th Troop Carrier Squadron War Diary," including "Squadron Medical Journal" (unpublished manuscript, 1941-1945), accessed via

Air Force Historical Research Agency, Maxwell Air Force Base, Montgomery, Alabama.

4. "April 1945," in "50th Troop Carrier Squadron War Diary," including "Squadron Medical Journal" (unpublished manuscript, 1941-1945), accessed via Air Force Historical Research Agency, Maxwell Air Force Base, Montgomery, Alabama.

Chapter Eleven

1. "April 1945," in "50th Troop Carrier Squadron War Diary," including "Squadron Medical Journal" (unpublished manuscript, 1941-1945), accessed via Air Force Historical Research Agency, Maxwell Air Force Base, Montgomery, Alabama.

Chapter Twelve

1. "May 1945," in "50th Troop Carrier Squadron War Diary," including "Squadron Medical Journal" (unpublished manuscript, 1941-1945), accessed via Air Force Historical Research Agency, Maxwell Air Force Base, Montgomery, Alabama.

2. Ibid.

3. Ibid., "June 1945."

4. Gale R. Ammerman, *An American Glider Pilot's Story: 81st Troop Carrier Squadron, 436th Troop Carrier Group* (Bennington, Vermont: Merriam Press, 2001).

Bibliography

"50th Troop Carrier Command War Diary," including "Squadron Medical Journal." Air Force Historical Research Agency, 1941-1945.

"71st SOS, Wings, Groups, Squadrons." Accessed April 28, 2007. http://www.71stsos.com.

Ammerman, Gale R. *An American Glider Pilot's Story*. Bennington, VT: Merriam Press, 2001.

Armfield, Blanch B. "Medical Department, United States Army in World War II." Edited by John Boyd Coates, Jr., and Charles M. Wiltse. Under the direction of Leonard D. Heaton. Washington, DC: Office of the Surgeon General, Department of the Army: 1963. Accessed May 14, 2011. http://history.amedd.army.mil/booksdocs/wwii/orgadmin/org_admin_wwii_chpt4.htm.

Belmont, Larry M. "The Cigarette Camps: US Army Camps in the Le Havre Area." Accessed April 30, 2008. http://www.skylighters.org/special/cigcamps/cigintro.html.

"Buchenwald and Dachau Concentration Camps." JewishGen. Accessed July 21, 2006. http://www.jewishgen.org.

Bunting, Edward. *WWII: Day by Day*. London: Dorling Kindersley Limited, 1990.

Bramble, Robert G. *History of the 50th Troop Carrier Squadron, 314th Troop Carrier Group, World War II*. Complied by group historian, assembled and audited.

"C-47." Cavanaugh Flight Museum. Accessed March 6, 2005. http://www.cavanaughflightmuseum.com.

Callahan, Robert E. *Mannheim to Landsberg: Six Horrendous Concentration Camps.* Accessed April 25, 2008. http://www.nuspel.org/rem5.html.

"Catalogue of the School of Medicine, Announcement for 1940-1941." *Bulletin of Vanderbilt University,* 40, no.9 (July 1940).

Cate, J. L. and Craven, W. F., eds. *The Army Air Forces in WWII.* Hyperwar, 2011. http://www.ibiblio.org/hyperwar/AAF/VII/AAF-VII-13.html.

Custis, Donald L. "Military Medicine for WWII to Vietnam." *Journal of the American Medical Association,* 264, no.17 (1990): 2259-2262. doi:10.1001/jama.1990.03450170107031.

"Doctors: WWII 1941-45." Army Air Corps Living History Group. Accessed July 2014. http://www.armyaircorps.us/Doctors.

Elie, Patrick. "D-Day: Normandy 1944-US Airborne in Cotentin." Accessed April 10, 2005. www.6juin1944.com/assault/aeropus/en_9tcc.php.

"Flight Surgeon's Handbook." US Government Printing Office: 1943.

Franklin, Robert. *Medic! How I fought WWII with Morphine, Sulfa and Iodine Swabs.* Lincoln, NE: Bison Books, 2006.

Gaillard, Jr., Ernest. *Flight Surgeon: Complete and Unabridged Combat Medical Diary, US Eighth Army Air Forces, 381st Bomb Group, 242nd Medical Dispensary, Station 167.* Edited and compiled by William N. Gaillard. Bloomington, IN: 1st Books Library, 2003.

Goldblatt, Gary. "Medical Detachment Diary, Index/242med, June 1943, Station #167." Accessed May 2013. Last updated March 25, 2014. http://www.cbi-history.com/part_iv_med.html.

Harkiewicz, Joseph. "Daily Chronicles of a USAAF Unit in England for the Invasion of Europe." Edited by Lewis E. Johnston. Air Mobility Command Museum. Accessed March 6, 2005. http://www.amcmuseum.org/history/wwii/daily_chronicles.php.

Harwood, Raymond. "9th US Air Force, Mission Procedures." Buddies of the Ninth Association. Accessed April 16, 2005. http://www.publicenquiry.co.uk.

Haulman, Daniel L. "Ninth Air Force (Air Forces Central) (ACC)." Air Force Historical Research Agency. Accessed April 10, 2005. Last Updated January 2, 2013. http://www.afhra.af.mil/factsheets/factsheet.asp?id=16122.

Herbert, Jr., William C. *Combat Surgeon*. Spartanburg, SC: Honoribus, 1993.

Hughey, Michael John. "Organization and Function of Army Medical Department Combat Stress Control Units." Operational Medicine 2001, Field Manual No. 22-51, Booklet 1. Accessed January 25, 2011. http://brooksidepress.org/Products/OperationalMedicine/DATA/operationalmed/Manuals.

"Invaders: The Story of the 50th Troop Carrier Wing." Lone Sentry. Accessed April 26, 2005. http://www.lonesentry.com/gi_stories_booklets/50thtroopcarrier.

Jervey, Jr., Harold E. "Memoires of WWII." U.S. National Library of Medicine. Accessed January 2011. http://www.nlm.nih.gov/hmd/oral_history/musc2.html.

Keyserling G. B. Herbert. "Navy Doctor." U.S. National Library of Medicine. Accessed September 24, 2010. http://www.nlm.nih.gov/hmd/oral_history/musc2.html#.

Monahan, Evelyn and Rosemary Neidel-Greenlee. *And If I Perish: Frontline U.S. Army Nurses in World War II.* New York: Alfred A. Knopf, 2002.

Moore, Samuel T. *Flight Surgeon: With the 81st Fighter Group in WWII.* With James Edwin Alexander. Oklahoma City: Macedon, 1999.

Nanney, James S. "Aeromedical Challenges in Mounting an Attack From Great Britain," in "Army Air Forces Medical Services in World War II." Air Force History and Museums Program, 1998. Accessed April 8, 2005. http://www.afhso.af.mil/shared/media/document/AFD-100923-014.pdf.

"Neil Robertson Stretcher." Integrated Publishing. Accessed December 12, 2010. http://navyadvancement.tpub.com/12018/css/12018_490.htm.

"People remember WWII nurses." US Air Force. Accessed April 23, 2008. http://www.af.mil/news/story.asp?storyID=123007904.

Piersall, Mark. "Air Medals." Accessed April 28, 2010. http://www.marksmedals.com.

"Processing of Patients, WWII Air Evacuation, Kits of Military Aircraft," WW2 US Medical Research Center. Accessed September 20, 2006. http://www.med-dept.com/terms.php.

Pyle, Ernie. *Brave Men.* New York: Grosset & Dunlop, 1943.

"Reunion Book." Vanderbilt University School of Medicine,

Class of 1941: 1991.

Rust, Kenn C. *The 9th Air Force in World II.* Falbrook, CA: Aero, 1967.

Sajna, Mike. "Medical School Graduate complies history of Pitt trained doctors' contribution in WWII." *University Times,* 29, no. 14 (March 20, 1997). Accessed March 16, 2012. http://www.pitt.edu/utimes/issues. www.mac10. umc.pitt.edu.

Sherman, Samuel Robert. "Oral Histories of WWII: Navy Flight Surgeon on USS Franklin" In "Oral Histories— Attacks on Japan, 1945." Naval History and Heritage Command. Accessed April 23, 2008. http://www. history.navy.mil.

Steinert, David. "World War II Combat Medic: Equipment of a WWII Combat Medic, The History of WWII Medical Equipment Stock List Numbers." Accessed April 23, 2006. http://home.att.net/~steinert/nepage2.htm.

Truman, Robert. "Control Towers in the UK, USAF, 9th Air Force." Accessed July 7, 2014. http://www. controltowers.co.uk.

"Wartime Airfield Accidents." WW2Talk. Accessed April 10, 2005. http://ww2talk.com/forums/topic/20012-wartime-airfield-accidents.

Wolfe, Martin. *Green Light: A Troop Carrier Squadron's War From Normandy to the Rhine.* University of Pennsylvania Press, 1989; repr., Washington, DC: Center for Air Force History, 1993.

Young, Charles D. "Historical Overview." Accessed April 26, 2005. http://www.usaaftroopcarrier.com/historical-overview/.

Index